1 Minute Wellness Messages

Quick Wellness Tips for Busy People

Dr. S. Don Kim

The purpose of this book is not to dispense medical
advice or prescribe the use of any technique as a form
of treatment for physical, emotional, or medical problems without the advice of a physician, either directly or
indirectly. The intent of the author is only to offer information of a general nature to help in a quest for physical, emotional and spiritual well-being. The author and
publisher assume no responsibility for results of actions
when using any information contained in this book for
personal healing.

Book Front Cover Design by KillerCovers - www.killercov-
ers.com | Book Back Cover Design by Dan Yeager - www.
nu-images.com | Interior Design by D.L. Hughes - www.
BookPublishingMentor.com | Illustrations Compiled by
Lainee Richards and Sandy Richards | Contributions and
Editing by Kara Tornquist | See page 281 for additional
credits.

ISBN: 978-0-9819628-1-8

A Note from Dr. Kim...

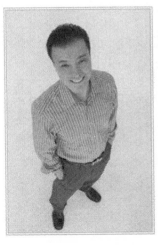

We are all incredibly busy and focused on running our daily lives. We spend most of our minutes each day taking care of others. Our work, home and family come first and we often forget to take care of ourselves. These messages are reminders to take just a minute every day to focus on your own health and wellness. You have the power to transform your life and be a healthier, happier you. You can form new health habits by making small painless changes, one day, one hour, and one minute at a time.

I believe that empowering education is the key to a prosperous and balanced life. It is my hope that you will be so inspired by these 1 Minute Wellness Messages that you will act on them and become healthier and happier.

Express Your Love Today!

Check Your Feet

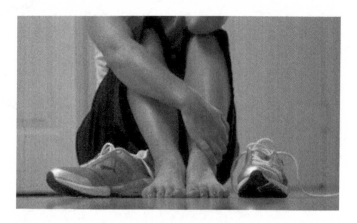

When you have sore knees, stiff hips or a painful lower back, you should have your feet checked. Flat feet can cause knocked knees, tilted hips and flattened backs.* Your feet are the foundation of your entire body, and if they're not stable, you could develop many health problems. Your feet are like tires of your car; if your tires get flat, you can't go anywhere!

Today, make an appointment with a foot doctor to get your feet checked if you have any of the above symptoms. Keep your tires pumped up!

Double Your Water

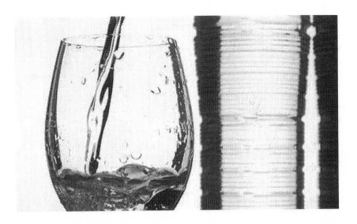

Your human body is 70% water, but some parts of the body contain even more: your cells are 90% water; your brain, 85%; your blood stream, 83%; your muscles, 75%; your joint cartilage, 82%; and your stomach lining is an amazing 98% water! You need to keep water flowing through your body daily to stay healthy. Dehydration is by far the number one cause of disease and cell death.*

Today, keep bottled water with you at all times and try to double your consumption. If you usually drink one bottle, today's the day to drink two.

A Handful of Calcium

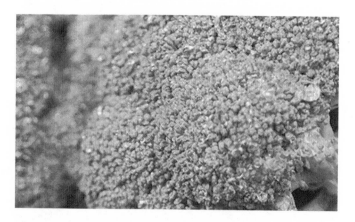

Calcium makes up more than 50% of your body's mineral content. Yet, surprisingly, more than 75% of Americans have calcium deficiencies.* Calcium is crucial for healthy teeth, strong bones, a powerful heart and regular muscle functions. Green leafy vegetables, nuts and seeds are great sources of abundant calcium.

Snack on a handful of steamed broccoli, raw almonds, or raw sunflower seeds today to get the calcium you need!

Dr. S. Don Kim

Eat Green Blood

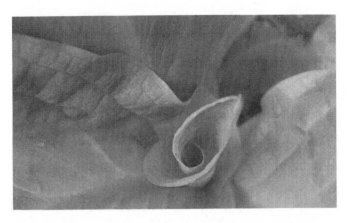

Did you know you lose about 2.4 million red blood cells every second of your life? That's about 25 trillion red blood cells every 120 days, which your body must replenish in order to keep you alive. Plants contain a pigment called chlorophyll, which is almost identical in structure to hemoglobin, a central part of red blood cell structure.*

Today, eat more green vegetables to replenish the huge loss of red blood cells you'll experience. Making sure that a large part of your plate is green at each meal contributes to healthy body, every day!

Fewer Legs the Better

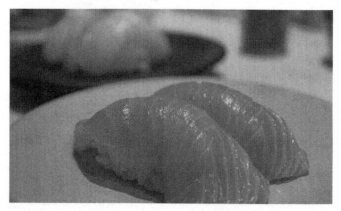

Meats from four-legged animals, such as beef, lamb, and pork, have the highest amount of saturated fats. Two-legged animals, like chicken and turkey, have less saturated fat, and no-legged critters like fish or tree foods such as nuts and seeds have the least amount of bad fats.*

Have more food with fewer legs, today. Choose fish, nuts and seeds over two or four-legged animals.

Microwaving Kills

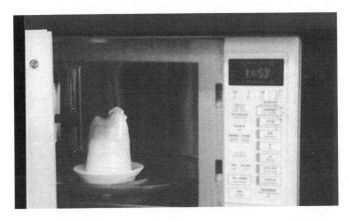

When food temperatures rise very fast, as with microwaving, all the valuable vitamins, minerals, enzymes and proteins are denatured and destroyed.

Research shows that microwave cooking is linked to cancer, which caused Russia to recently ban micro-waving throughout the whole country!*

Use steaming, boiling, baking or broiling when heating food for you and your family and avoid the harmful effects of microwaves.

Pebble in Your Foot

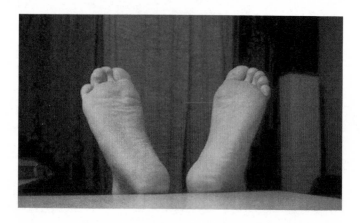

Did you know that there are 250,000 sweat glands in your foot?*   When you develop callous tissues under the foot, the sweat cannot get through. Instead, the sweat goes back into the foot and hardens like a cyst. This is called *porokeratosis*. This is very painful and patients describe this condition as feeling as if they have a "pebble" in their foot.

Today, check your feet to see if you have callous tissues. Make sure you eliminate the cause of these callous tissues. If you already have pebbles in your feet, these can be frozen off easily by your foot doctor.

When Not to Drink

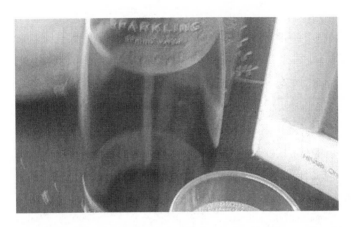

Most people eat their meals too fast. They don't chew their food sufficiently, so they end up drinking fluid to wash it down. But when you have a beverage with food, your digestive enzymes become diluted, your meal doesn't break down completely, and you end up storing the food as fat.* You should drink ~~30 minutes before~~ and ~~30 minutes after~~ the eating, but not during a meal.

Reduce the amount of water or other beverages during your meals today. If you can't cut out a beverage completely, try sipping it instead of drinking fully.

How Colorful is Your Plate?

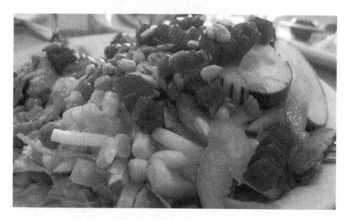

Phytonutrients are biological substances that give fruits and vegetables their color, flavor, smell and disease resistance. There are an estimated 40,000 phytonutrients available in colorful foods, and they can prevent cancer, heart disease, arthritis, infection, allergies and numerous other diseases.*

Look down at your plate today when you're eating. It should look like a colorful painting. Try to make your plate more vibrant with fresh fruits and vegetables at every meal.

Friendly Probiotics

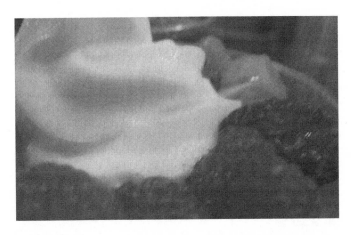

We have more than 100 trillion bacteria living in our intestines, many of which are "friendly" *probiotics* that break down our food. These helpful bacteria also strengthen your immune system, remove toxins from your body and create B vitamins.* Foods rich in probiotics include sauerkraut, soy sauce, Kimchi and organic yogurt.

Eat some probiotic-rich foods today for better bowel health. If you don't like any of the foods listed above, make sure you take a supplement with at least 10 billion probiotics in it.

Help Your
Shock Absorbers

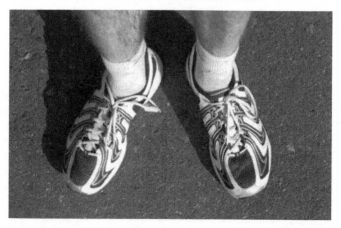

From the moment you put your first foot in front of the other to walk, your feet become shock absorbers. Feet flex to reduce the pressure of your weight from the ground's reactive forces. When you are walking, you put at least double of your weight per step. When you are running, you can load up to three times of your weight per step!*

Help your foot by wearing soft-heeled shoes and reduce your weight to unload the pressure to the steps. This will reduce the breakdown of your foot.

Dr. S. Don Kim

Processed, Dead Salt Kills

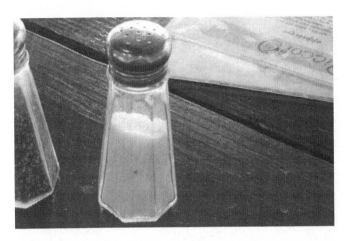

Much of the salt sold in grocery stores has been processed and bleached with chemicals, hence its white color. This is done to lengthen its shelf-life and improve its appearance and consistency. Unfortunately, this processing removes crucial minerals and devitalizes the salt.* Dead, processed salt dehydrates cells and eventually leads to cell deaths. Real, natural salt, on the other hand, is pink, grey, purple and other colors because minerals are still a vibrant part of it.

Replace processed white salt with natural colorful salt today. Cook only with the colorful salts from now on.

"~~Walking~~ is Man's Best Medicine" - Hippocrates

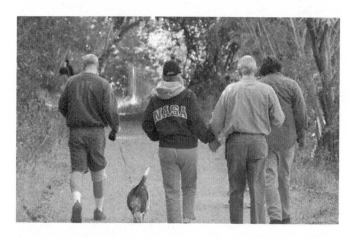

Walking is an easy aerobic exercise. It is safe, inexpensive, convenient and requires no training or equipment. Walking leads to better breathing, stronger immunity, increased muscular strength, improved balance and flexibility, stronger bones, better sleep and less depression.* Most importantly, the rhythmic motion of walking synchronizes your brain waves, leading to a calmer state and reduced stress.

Take a walking break for five minutes today. Instead of having a sit-down meeting in your office, try a walking meeting outside. How did you feel?

Power Naps Anyone?

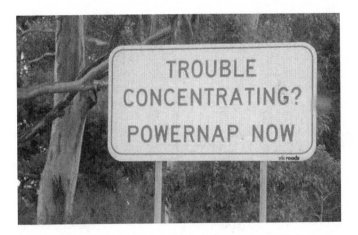

In many countries around the world, people take a nap every afternoon. Really! All the stores and businesses shut down for a few hours so people can take naps. Siestas make sense because we are actually designed to sleep twice a day. Taking naps is proven to increase alertness and enhance performance throughout the day.*Based on the rhythm of life, our bodies usually need naps between 2 and 3 p.m.

Take a power nap today for 10 to 20 minutes. Notice your energy surge after the nap. You may want to do it again tomorrow.

Eating Under Stress

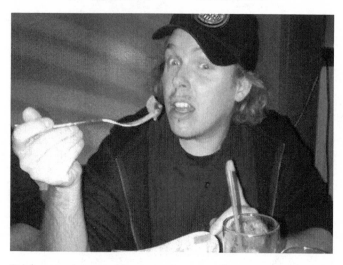

Did you know that eating under stress could slow down your metabolism and make you gain weight? Your meal becomes stressful when you eat it too fast, don't chew enough, foster guilt about your food, eat when you're upset and don't breathe while eating. Any of these behaviors will decrease nutrient absorption and increase your cholesterol levels, triglyceride levels and salt retention while bringing on many more negative effects.*

Today, relax while eating by slowing down and enjoying your food. Take three deep breaths before your meals to help calm yourself.

Dr. S. Don Kim

Vacate Your Mind

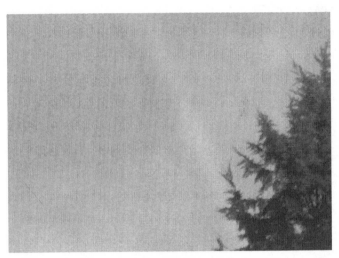

Most of us are bombarded with more than 5,000 different advertisement messages every day.* These ads are from news-papers, TV, radio, the Internet, billboards, magazines, cell phones and other places. They crowd our minds and over-burden our thoughts. Taking a break, such as News "fasts", TV "fasts" and computer "fasts" are all good ways to clear your mind of unnecessary negativity.

Fast from some form of technology that usually consumes your day. Try no news, no TV or no internet for a day!

Dangers of Sitting

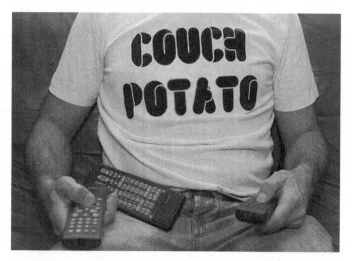

Americans sit in the car, at a desk, in front of TVs and computers then spend endless hours playing video games. We can sit up to ten hours a day with these activities.* Sitting creates tight hamstrings and hip flexors. This in turn can cause tilted pelvis and eventual back pain. In other words, too much sitting causes back pain.

Today count the number of hours you sit each day. Then reduce your sitting activities in half. Take a break from endless TV channel and internet surfing. How does your back feel at the end of the day?

An Old Friend

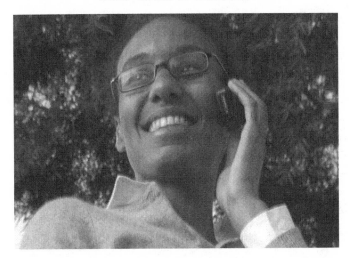

Are you feeling a little down today? Do you feel that you are not appreciated? Are you stressed out? Do you feel stuck? Is something irritating you?

Reconnecting with old friends is a good remedy for boredom, and it will lift up your spirit. Revisiting an old friendship will definitely get you out of your current state.*

Call an old friend out of the blue today; you will feel revitalized afterward!

Toxic Sunscreens

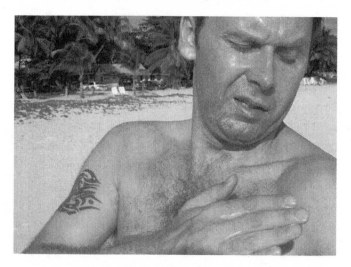

Toxic chemicals in sunscreens can cause skin cancer. Octyl-dimethyl-PABA (OD – PABA), Benzophenone-3 (Bp-3), Homosalate (HMS), Octyl-methoxycinnamate (OMC) and 4-methyl-benzylidene camper (4-MBC) are all toxic chemicals commonly found in sun block products. The sun does not cause skin cancer, but these toxic sunscreens do.*

From now on, use natural sunscreens with vitamins C and E included. Apply zinc oxide to places that burn easily. Of course, avoid direct sunlight for long periods, too.

Just Laugh

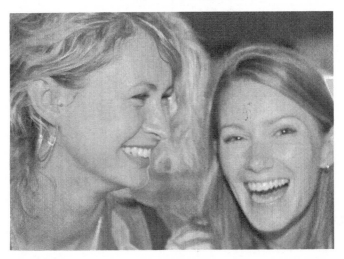

The human race has only one really effective weapon, and that is laughter. The moment it arises, all your irritations and resentments slip away and the sunny spirit takes their place.

Actively look for things to laugh about today, then laugh as much as you can.

Express Your Love

There are many ways to express your love to others. You can write love letters, send flowers, cook a delicious meal, give hugs, offer your assistance on a big project, volunteer to help others in need, say kind words, give undivided attention, listen, spend quality time, cuddle, give a massage or buy gifts.

Express your feelings to someone you love by doing one of the things listed above today, even if that person is yourself!

MSG Makes you Sick and Fat

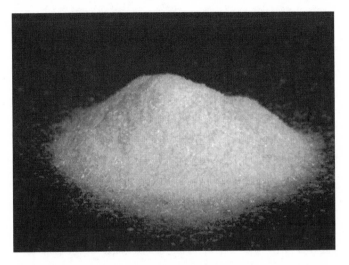

MSG (monosodium glutamate) is an extremely toxic food taste enhancer. It is an *excitotoxin* that makes your cells overexcited and causes them to fire uncontrollably, which eventually causes cell death. MSG can lead to autism, schizophrenia, seizures, brain tumors, Alzheimer's disease, cerebral palsy, episodic violence and criminal behaviors. MSG will also increase your appetite and make you gain weight.*

Read the labels of food products to avoid toxic MSG. If you become extremely thirsty after you eat at a restaurant, watch out!

Most Undertreated Medical Problem

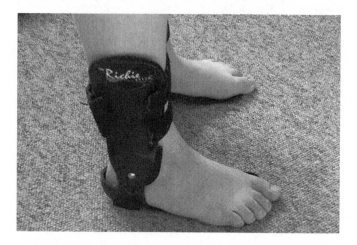

Journal of American Medical Association states that the ankle sprain is the most under treated medical problem of all time.* Most people under treat the ankle sprains with just icing, ace bandage or sometimes crutches. This is just not enough for most of the ankle sprains, especially the ones with loud noise during the sprain, instant bruising and extreme swelling.

If you sprain your ankle severely, you need to immobilize it aggressively either with a boot or a cast. You need to see your foot doctor immediately for an X-ray and treatment. You don't want residual problems that may require surgical intervention.

Reverse your Shrinking

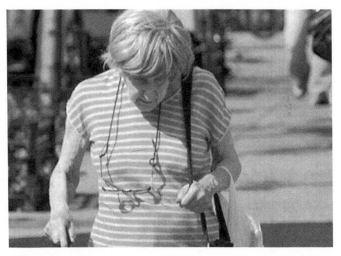

You've probably heard that people shrink as they get older, which is true. Many people suffer from rickets, a vitamin D deficiency that causes bowed legs and a hunched body. You can take all the calcium you want, but unless you get vitamin D from sunlight, the calcium will not get into your bones. Sunlight can prevent and even reverse osteoporosis and rickets.*

Get outside and get some sun today! Enjoy outdoor activities like picnics, games, sports, a hike or just take a walk around your neighborhood. Your health depends on it!

Endorphins, The Elixir of Life

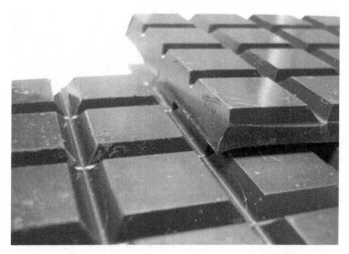

Endorphins are produced within our bodies and are 200 times stronger than the pain killer morphine. In fact, the word "endorphin" is derived from "endogenous morphine." Endorphins kill pain, create pleasure, boost our immune systems, and activate our natural killer cells that can fight cancer cells. And, they have no side effects!*

Let's help our bodies produce endorphins today. Did you know that some of the most pleasurable things can boost endorphins? Laugh out loud, have a chiropractic adjustment, get an acupuncture treatment, enjoy a deep tissue massage or eat dark chocolate (not milk chocolate) to get your natural painkillers flowing. Wow!

Citrus Fruit

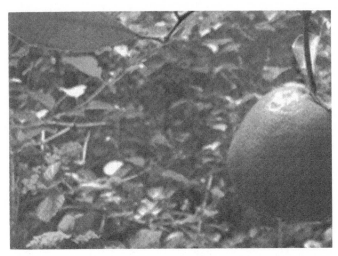

Oranges, grapefruits and other citrus fruits look similar to female mammary glands. Interestingly, they can improve breast health and facilitate the movement of lymphatic fluid in and out of the breasts. These fruits are also full of vitamin C — a powerful antioxidant that fights all forms of disease — from the common cold to cancer and everything in between.*

Have oranges or grapefruits as snacks today to boost your citrus intake. To get the full benefit, make sure you eat the white pith, as it contains most of the citrus fruits' Vitamin C!

Celebrate Your Meals

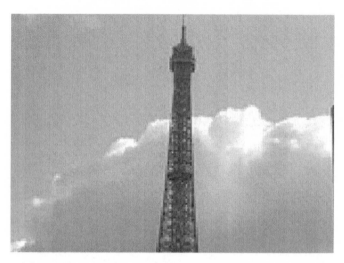

Did you know that celebrating your meals could increase your metabolism and help you lose weight? Think about French people, who are known to truly celebrate all of their meals. They consume just as much as food as Americans, but they don't get fat because they take their time and enjoy eating. This is known as the "French paradox."* When you feel pleasure in your food, your endorphins kick in to pump up your metabolic rate.

When you have your meals today, try to experience the food; touch it, savor it, notice it, smell it and ponder its color. Enjoy your food for better health!

Break Your Fast

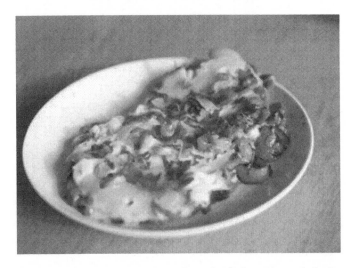

Each morning, you need to break your nightly fast with a long, robust, sit-down breakfast. Numerous studies show that thin, healthy people eat breakfast every morning.* You set the tone for the rest of your day with what you eat for breakfast. For the best health and the best metabolism, you need a protein-rich breakfast complete with plenty of fruits and vegetables.

The first step is to commit to eat something for breakfast. But for the very best health, include vegetable juice, fresh seasonal fruits, organic cage-free eggs, salads (yes, for breakfast!), protein shakes or vegetable soup in your morning meal.

Prevent Ankle Sprains

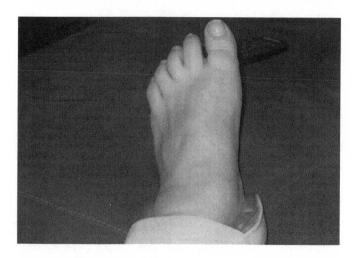

An ankle sprain is one of the most common sports injuries. There are three ligaments that hold the out-step of the ankle joint. However, there are five ligaments holding the instep of the ankle joint. This imbalance causes over 90% of sprains to the outstep of the ankle.

When you are engaged in high impact sports such as basketball, football, volleyball and racquetball, use an ankle brace. An ankle brace is known to increase your *proprioceptive* senses to trigger preventative action of the muscles.*

Forgive Someone Today

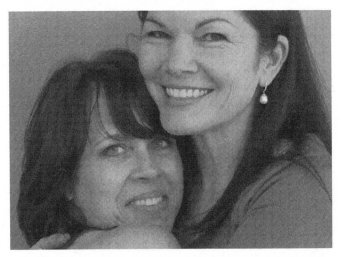

Forgiveness is freedom. When you forgive, you free yourself from self-inflicted bondage. In other words, you must forgive others to help yourself. Most of the time, when you are conflicted about someone who hurt you, the other person doesn't even realize that you are upset. You are not hurting anyone but yourself when you refuse to offer forgiveness.

Think of one person whom you can't forgive. Call, write or visit this person today if you can, but even if you can't, forgive them anyway.

Cry Your Way to Health

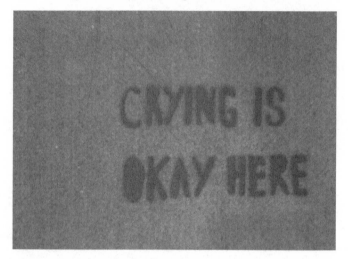

Tears are sometimes the most effective way to express your emotions. Crying is often triggered by anger and grief, but tears can also result from sadness, happiness, fear, laughter, frustration, remorse or other strong feelings. It is not healthy to hold back your tears. You need to let your tears flow to be emotionally healthy because crying eliminates emotional toxins.*

Have a crying session today. Watch a touching movie, have a deep conversation or participate in an inspirational service to allow your tears to flow and let the toxins go.

Diet Sodas

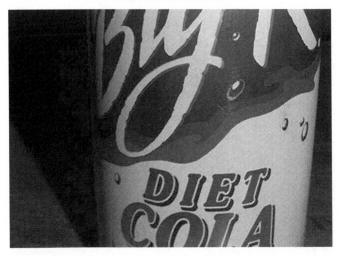

Aspartame, which is the artificial sweetener in almost all diet sodas, contains toxic methanol. Methanol breaks down into phenylalanine and aspartic acid, both of which can cause severe headaches, seizures, vision impairment, dizziness, rashes, extreme fatigue, depression, personality changes, confusion, memory loss, weight gain, diabetes and many other health problems. Aspartame is also in breakfast cereals and chewing gum. It is highly addicting and 200 times sweeter than sugar.*

Diet sodas don't help you manage your weight; they actually make you fat and sick. Let's stop drinking all diet sodas as of today.

Sweating

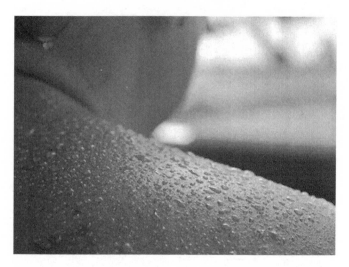

Minerals and other small, toxic particles are eliminated from your body when you sweat. Your skin is the largest organ of your body, and sweating is the most effective way to detoxify because of the sheer volume of sweat you produce. You will get the maximum benefit from this form of detoxification when you exercise and sweat on a regular basis.*

Break a sweat today. Exercise or engage in other physical activities or spend some time in an infrared sauna to detoxify through sweating.

High Fructose Corn Syrup

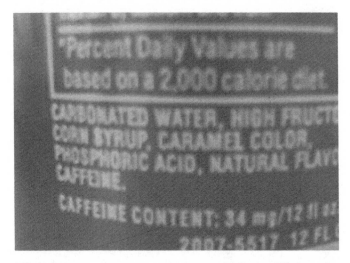

High fructose corn syrup is made from extremely processed corn products, and it's highly addictive and fattening. It is found in most packaged foods, regular sodas and beverages, ice cream, candy, jam, ketchup and baked goods. Consuming high fructose corn syrup leads to blood sugar problems, depression, fatigue, B-vitamin deficiency, hyperactivity, indigestion, tooth decay, periodontal disease and elevated triglyceride levels.*

Read the labels on packaged foods and sodas you consider buying today. If you see high fructose corn syrup on products, put them back on the shelf.

Prevent Ingrown Nails

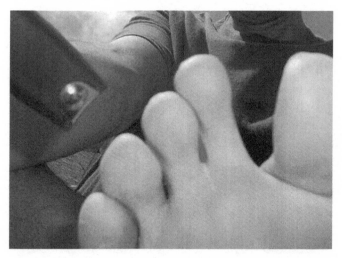

Ingrown nails are caused by cutting or digging the corners too short.* They can also come from wearing shoes that are too tight or small. Many people have fungus in their toenails and when you are infected with nail fungus, your nail will grow thick and grow improperly.

Cut your toenails straight across without going into the corners. Do not wear shoes too tight. You should also leave a thumb-sized space between your longest toe and the tip of your shoes. Treat any fungus in your nails.

Light and Social Dinner

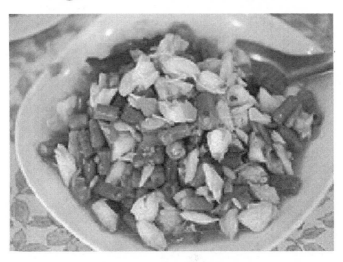

Dinner should be the smallest meal of your day. In the evening, you no longer need much fuel and your body virtually stops producing any digestive enzymes. A huge dinner will just sit in your stomach and doesn't get digested properly.* This is why many people are overweight—they eat too much food too late at night!

Safeguard your health by reducing the size of your dinner dramatically today. Keep your dinner light and social.

Pray for Healing

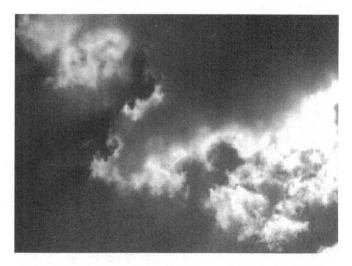

Matter can be controlled and directed by thought, and this power can be harnessed by prayer and used to heal. We are all creators, and we are constantly creating good and bad things through the use or misuse of our thought power. If we visualize our goals and believe in them, we will reach them. Every thought is a prayer, and our prayers give us healing energy.

Pray for your own healing today. When you're healthy you can help others even more, maybe you'll even be an answer to someone else's prayers.

Walnut Brain

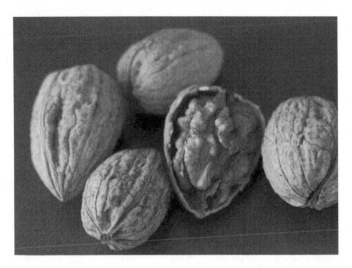

Have you ever noticed that a walnut looks like a little brain, with a left and right hemisphere, an upper cerebrum and a lower cerebellum? The wrinkles and folds on the nut are even similar to the brain's neo-cortex. Appropriately, walnuts help brain function.*

Improving your memory and cognition is as easy as enjoying a healthy meal or snack that includes a serving of walnuts.

Female Avocados

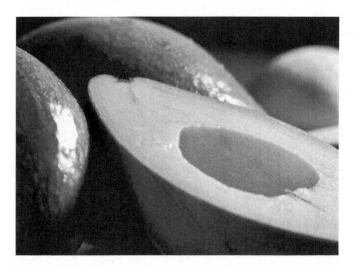

The nutrients found in avocados help a woman's cervix and uterus stay healthy; the fruits even look a bit like these organs. Avocados can also balance female hormones and have been shown to prevent cervical cancer.* And how profound is this: It takes exactly nine months to grow an avocado from blossom to ripened fruit!

Avocados taste great and can be enjoyed in a salad, as a guacamole dip or on a sandwich. They're good for men too!

How to be Happy

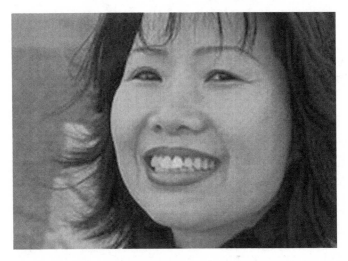

You will be happy when: you find meaning and purpose in your life, when you don't lose sight of your goals, when you find the positive in every situation, when you seek to do good no matter what, and when you find good people and keep them around you.

Be happy today by practicing one of the things above.

Increase Your Steps

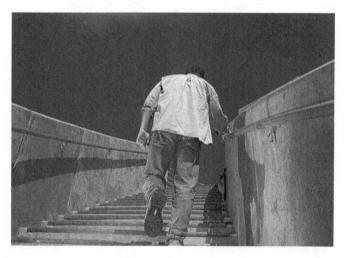

The majority of Americans walk fewer than 2,000 steps each day, which is less than one mile. It is well known that you need to walk at least 10,000 steps—or five miles—a day to stay healthy.* Walking the recommended amount takes about one hour and forty minutes. You need to increase your number of steps to stay healthy.

Today, walk up the stairs instead of taking elevators or escalators. Park farther away and walk to stores or your office rather than fighting for the closest spot.

You Must Supplement

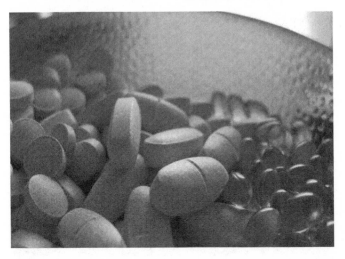

Over the past 100 years, soil quality around the world has been leached of its vital mineral content. North American soils are the worst of all, with 85% of natural minerals depleted. When you eat foods that are grown in such depleted soils, you do not get enough nutrients.* You must supplement vitamins and minerals daily since it has become virtually impossible to get essential nutrients through your diet alone.

Start the habit of taking vitamin and mineral supplements today. Try to find natural or organic supplement brands that used food-based ingredients.

Gouty Attack!

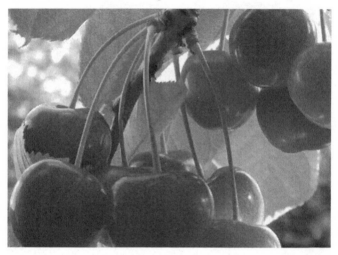

Gout is an extremely painful arthritic condition that most commonly attacks your big toe joint. Ninety five percent of the time, gout attacks middle-aged men who eat a lot of meat and drink alcohol.* Colchicine and Indocin are the main medications to combat gout, but they are riddled with side effects of upset stomach, hair loss, depression and liver toxicity to name a few.

Decrease consumption of high protein diet of organ meat, anchovies, dried beans, fish and mushrooms. Reduce alcohol and weight. Drink cherry juice and eat lot of cherries. Take supplements such as fish oil (EPA), vitamin E, folic acid, and celery seed extract.

Flush Your Nose

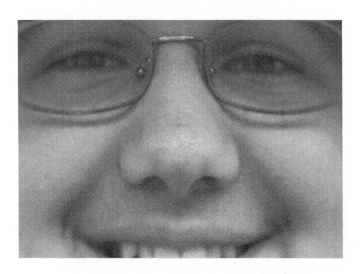

Do you feel a flu coming on? Do you have a stuffy nose? Are your sinuses bothering you? Try flushing your nose with natural salt to clear up these problems. Natural salt sinus flushes are very effective in fighting the flu, sinus infections, hay fever, sore throats, runny noses, bronchitis and asthma.* Especially during the flu season, sinus flushes can combat and prevent illness.

Try a sinus flush today using these methods: combine one-half cup warm water with one-half teaspoon of natural salt. Inhale the salt water into each of your nostrils, one at a time, and spit the liquid out though your mouth. You will notice your nose clearing up right away!

The Incredible Benefits of Salt Lamps

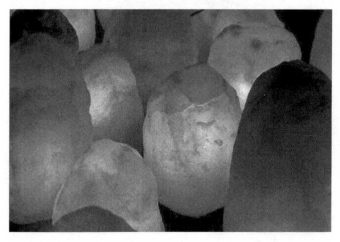

Salt lamps are powerful ways to detoxify your homes. The average American spends 65 to 90 percent of their life indoors, and inside environments can be five times more polluted than outdoor ones! Salt lamps emit negatively charged ions to decrease indoor pollutants like bacteria, fungi, pollen, dust mites, animal dander and mold. They are natural air purifiers and ionizers that don't require a large up-front investment or costly filter replacements.*

Get a salt lamp today. They not only look great but also have many health benefits for your indoor environment.

Electromagnetic Pollution

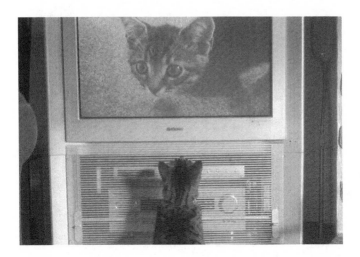

TVs and computers produce electromagnetic vibrations at a frequency of around 100 to 160 hertz. In comparison, our brain waves vibrate at 8 hertz. That means our bodies are regularly exposed to frequencies that are 20 times higher than those of our brains! This can lead to problems with concentration, nervousness, insomnia and even cancer.*

Make an effort to reduce the time you spend in front of the TV or computer today. Take frequent breaks while using your computer, and don't keep it on unless you are using it.

Declutter

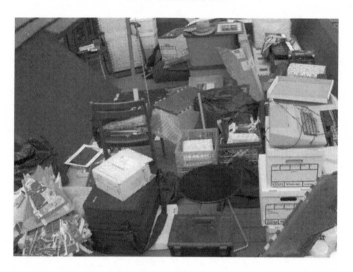

Have you ever noticed that you need to vacate your personal space of extra stuff often? How does it pile up so quickly? Eliminating unnecessary clutter from your closet, garage, kitchen, office, back yard and bedroom will help you feel better. Clearing these spaces will give you a sense of freedom and control. Decluttering not only vacates your physical space, but it also helps clear your mind.

Pick one of your personal spaces to declutter today. Enjoy!

Contrast Baths

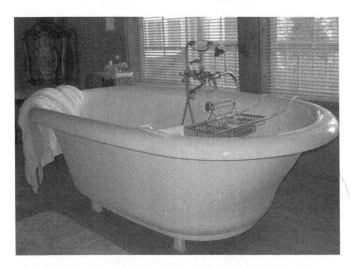

When you alternate hot and cold during your shower, it stimulates circulation and your immune system. This process is called contrast bathing or hydrotherapy, and is an effective way to detoxify your body.* Yogis have been practicing this for thousands of years. Contrast bathing is based on the principle that by alternately contracting and dilating the blood vessels through the varying water temperature, circulation is improved and the removal of waste products is accelerated. If you belong to a gym or health club, you can alternate sauna and cold plunge or shower to feel energized.

Take a contrast bath today and notice how invigorated you feel.

Over-rated Cotton Socks

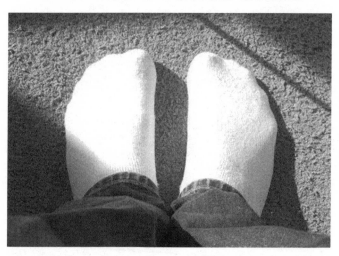

Cotton is a natural fiber, which absorbs and retains moisture, often causing the skin to become macerated and wrinkled--just like what happens to the skin when it is submerged in a pool or bathtub for a long time.* Wet skin is more likely to form blisters, which is why cotton socks should be avoided.

Wear acrylic or synthetic socks that don't retain moisture. These socks wick away moisture from your foot and help keep them dry and healthy.

Jump Your Way to Health

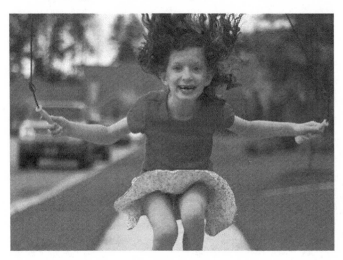

As a kid you were probably told never to jump on the bed. But, jumping is actually good for you! Jump on a rebounder or trampoline for 3-5 minutes at a time. This shakes up your whole body and stimulates the lymphatic system, which carries nutrients to every cell in your body and takes waste products away. If you don't have a rebounder, try jump roping or "jumping jacks" instead. Jumping is reported to increase lymph flow by 15 to 30 times.*

Use a rebounder or jump for 3-5 minutes today. How did you feel? Increase your daily jumping time as you can tolerate more.

Vanadium for Diabetes

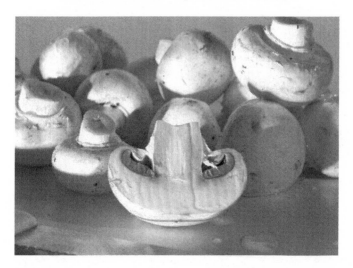

The single most effective weapon for managing blood sugar is vanadium. Vanadium is a trace mineral that works like insulin to increase the amount of glucose and amino acids driven into muscle tissue. This helps to balance blood sugar levels and aids in the release of energy. Vanadyl sulfate is a compound of vanadium, sulfur and oxygen and is the most effective form of vanadium for diabetes. You need about 100mg per day, but make sure to consult with your physician before starting any treatment.*

If you want to improve sugar metabolism, try these foods in your diet: black pepper, dill seed, parsley, olives, olive oil, sunflower oil, apples, oats, radishes, mushrooms, soy and corn.

Accept the Differences

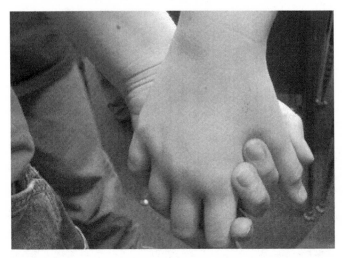

"What women want: To be loved, to be listened to, to be desired, to be respected, to be needed, to be trusted, and sometimes, just to be held. What men want: Tickets to the World Series." -- Dave Barry.

Accepting the fact that we are made differently will improve your relationships with others. You can get different needs met from the many people in your life. By expecting our spouse or partner to fulfill our every need, we set ourselves up for disappointment. As you realize that some things are better accomplished with some of the other people in your life, happiness and satisfaction can greatly improve.

Torment of Cholesterol Lowering Drugs

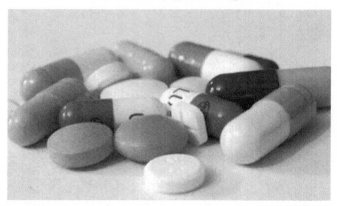

Thirty million Americans spent $34 billion on cholesterol lowering drugs in 2009.* These statin drugs such as, Vytorin, Lipitor and Crestor can create muscle pain, weakness, numbness, nerve damage, fatigue, shortness of breath, confusion, depression, hostility, sexual dysfunction and heart failure. These common drugs also drain your body out of CoQ10, which is an antioxidant that helps cells to produce *adenosine triphosphate*-the energy source of all cells.

Supplement with organic red yeast rice extract and CoQ10 to reverse this high cholesterol condition instead of taking statin drugs. Celery stalks have been known to decrease high cholesterol levels, too. Always consult with your physician before stopping or starting any medication.

Dr. S. Don Kim

Alternative Therapies for Pain

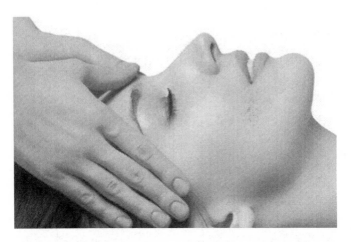

One third of Americans who suffer with chronic pain use an alternative therapy such as acupuncture, chiropractic, massage, magnet, herbalism, Ayurveda, meditation, yoga, biofeedback, hypnosis, homeopathy, nutrition and other therapies. Many of these treatments have been in use for thousands of years with a multitude of reported health benefits.

Try one of the alternative therapies to manage your pain. What did you like about that therapy?

Check Your Shoe Wear Pattern

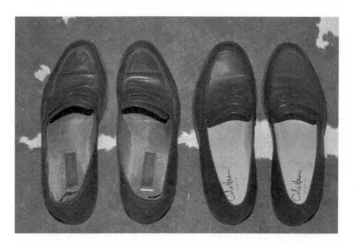

The wear pattern of a shoe often gives an indication of how the foot functions. Place the shoe on a table and look at the shoe at the back of the heel counter. If the top of the shoe excessively leans in toward the opposite foot, it is likely that your foot is flexible and flat. If the top of the shoe leans excessively away from the opposite foot, it is likely that the foot is too rigid and high arched.*

Check out your shoe wear pattern. If they are leaning dramatically toward either direction, you need to see a foot specialist right away.

Dr. S. Don Kim

Are You Deficient in Omega-3?

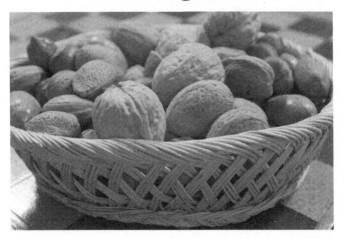

If you have high blood pressure, high choles-terol, aching or stiff joints, poor circulation, depression, dry eyes, dry skin or dry nails, you most likely are deficient in Omega-3 fats. According to the Harvard School of Public Health, this deficiency causes nearly 100,000 preventable deaths each year in the U.S. alone.*

Supplement at least 1,000 mg of fish or flaxseed oil every day. Choose organic cold pressed oils and increase your consumption of foods natu-rally high in Omega-3s such as pumpkin seeds, cabbage, walnuts, anchovies, halibut, salmon, tofu and cauliflower. Consult with your physi-cian before stopping or starting any medication.

Expect Nothing in Return

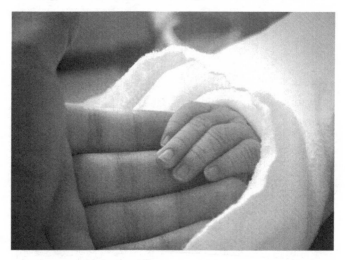

Expect nothing in return when it comes to relationships. Demonstrate respect, kindness and graciousness persistently. Even when others don't respond in kind, remember to expect nothing in return. This principle will transcend your relationships.

Pick a person whom you have hard time demonstrating respect and kindness. Just respect and be kind to this person without expecting the same in return. Watch what happens to the relationship.

Can You Remember?

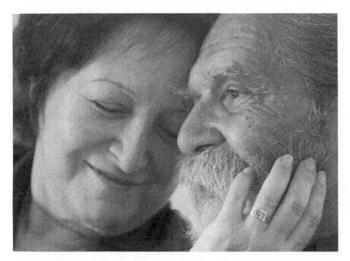

If you plan to live into your eighties, then your chances of suffering from Alzheimer's may be as high as fifty percent.* The common signs of early brain decay are slow recall, fuzzy memory, confusion with time, losing things, low mental energy and withdrawal from activities.

Supplement your diet with CoQ10, curcumin in curry spice, cherry and DHA (Omega-3 oil) to support a healthy memory. Always consult with your physician before stopping or starting any medication.

Help Others

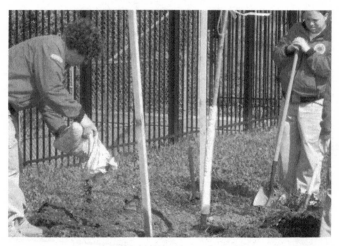

If you are not getting what you want in life, you may not be giving enough of yourself. Zig Zigler said, "You can have anything you want in life, if you will just help enough other people get what they want."

Look around to find someone who needs your help today. When you help others, you will benefit the most.

Dr. S. Don Kim

Miracles of Aloe Vera

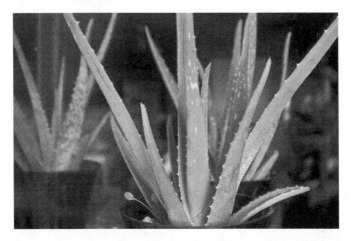

Aloe Vera has been used for thousands of years for medicinal purposes. It is commonly known for sunburn treatments, rash relief and fungicidal properties.* In addition, this miracle plant helps treat immune system diseases, anti-inflammatory diseases, menstrual cramps and digestive system disorders including irritable bowel syndrome. Aloe also holds moisture and adds flexibility to all seven layers of skin.

Growing aloe is quite easy; try growing a plant in your house or back yard. Use a knife to peel the skin from the hearty leaves and apply the gel on to your skin. Make juice out of the pulp inside of the leaves to enhance digestive function. Always consult with your physician before stopping or starting any medication.

Compression Socks

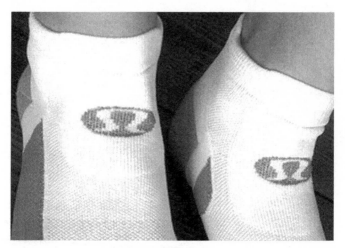

Compression socks have the greatest pressure at the ankle and sequentially less up the leg. They help conditions like swelling of the lower extremities, varicose veins, fatigue of the legs, blood clots, calf muscle cramps, tired, aching feet and legs, and lymph edema in the legs and feet.*

If you have any of the mentioned conditions, ask your doctor to prescribe compression socks.

Discipline

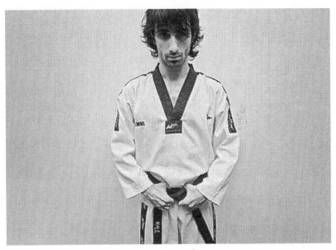

Discipline makes a difference between the good and the great. Discipline is a decision rather than a natural skill. It is the ability to stay the course and complete promises you have made for yourself and others. It's a habit and a self-fulfilling prophecy built into one. Once achieved, discipline builds confidence and self-esteem, which can make you believe that almost anything is possible (and it is!).

What area of your health do you lack discipline in: diet, exercise, rest or faith? Decide today to improve your discipline by scheduling your health activities. Then do it.

12 Pounds of Waste

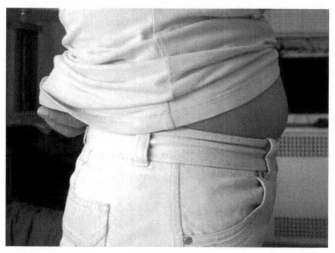

Americans store an average of twelve pounds of fecal waste in their colon. This comes from diets lacking enough fiber, over-processed and refined foods that become toxic, immovable and impacted in the colon. This can cause weight gain, headaches, backache, hemorrhoids, fatigue, insomnia, indigestion, allergies, abdominal discomfort, dry skin and in some cases, even cancer.*

Cleanse and detoxify your colon today with lots of water and green vegetables at every meal. Look down at your plate to make sure half of your plate is greens. Always consult with your physician before beginning a detoxification regimen.

Love Yourself

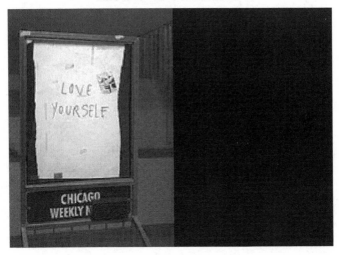

Everything starts with you. You can lovingly look at your family, society and even your country, but only truly, if you can look at yourself with love first. You may see yourself as unlovable; you need to learn to look at yourself with the eyes of love if for no other reason than because you are one of a kind in this world.

Learn to love yourself. If you don't, you won't be able to love anyone or anything else. This world doesn't exist without you.

Add This Spice

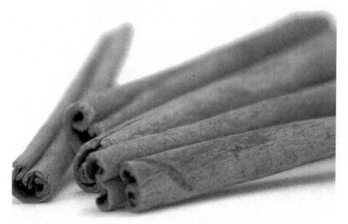

Cinnamon is a spice from the brown bark of the cinnamon tree and a well-known flavor ingredient in many foods. Research has found that one gram of cinnamon--less than half a teaspoon--promotes normal blood sugar levels. Cinnamon contains an ingredient called methylhydroxy chalcone polymer (MHCP), which is a potent antioxidant and also improves insulin sensitivity.* Cinnamon also has anti-clotting and anti-microbial properties and supports healthy brain and colon function.

Add this warm and nutritive spice to your diet to improve your health. Cinnamon is tasty sprinkled on toast or cereal and makes a great tea. You can add to curries and soups for an extra spicy flavor. Consult with your physician before stopping or starting any medication.

Gratitude

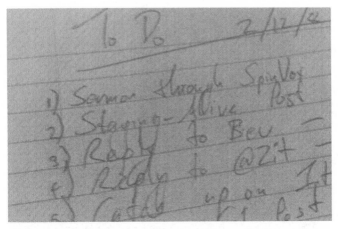

We all face adversity in our lives. It is not the adversity, but how we react to it that will determine the joy and happiness in our life. When you are going through life's trying times, rather than spending time feeling sorry for yourself, think of the things that you are thankful for. Soon the problems you face will not affect you as negatively.

List all the things that you are thankful for in your life. Start with your family and friends. This will lift your spirit to one of happiness and joy.

Shoe Fit Test

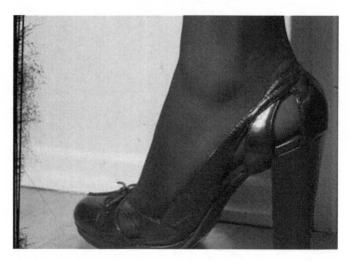

Did you know that two thirds of women wear shoes that are smaller than their feet?* This is the biggest self-inflicted trauma that people put themselves into in the name of fashion.

Stand barefoot on a blank piece of paper. Trace the outline of your foot. Then place your favorite shoe on top of this outline and draw over it. What do you see? Which is larger? Perform the above shoe fit test on your favorite shoes. How did you measure up?

Green Tea for Longevity

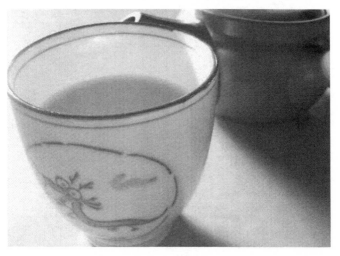

With an average life expectancy of 82, the Japanese live longer than anyone else in the world. The powerful antioxidant called EGCG in green tea is known to promote longevity. EGCG also protects heart health, helps manage weight, regulates blood sugar, reduces inflammation, boosts immunity and protects brain cells.*

Enjoy a cup of green tea today. Take time to enjoy the soothing aroma of the tea. Always consult with your physician before stopping or starting any medication.

Laugh At Yourself

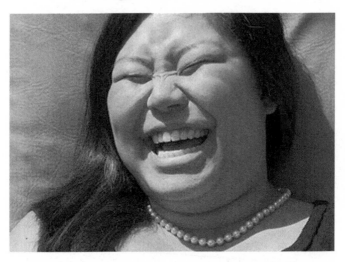

People take themselves too seriously. They live in their past failures, have low self-esteem and can't laugh at themselves. These are the reasons why people can't cope with life too well and become sick. You need to learn to laugh at your mistakes and failures. You need to realize that every master was once a disaster.

Find things about yourself to laugh at today. Whenever you make a mistake, just laugh!

Power of Resveratrol

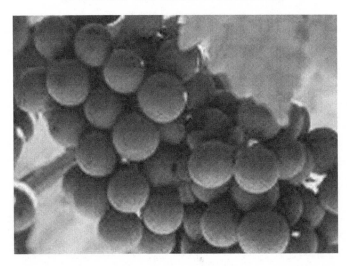

Resveratrol is a powerful antioxidant found in the skin of grapes that protects against the degenerative diseases of aging. Recent studies have revealed that it is one reason that cultures who consume a lot of red wine are healthier than those that don't. Resveratrol activates anti-aging genes, fights free radicals, helps manage weight, protects cardiovascular health, balances blood sugar levels, fights inflammation, supports healthy immunity and protects brain health.*

Add organic concord grapes, grapeskin extract, red wine or blueberries to your diet and enjoy the delicious taste of anti-aging!

Open Your Mind

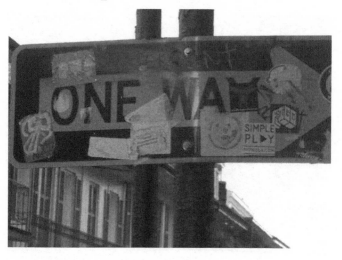

Always be on the lookout for "new" ways to do "old" things. Keep your mind open to using alternative methods and plans of action. This way you may find a better way to get twice much done in less than half of the time.

Take a different route home today. Ask yourself why you are doing certain things in a certain way. Do something differently than you normally do. How do you feel?

Are You Squeaky?

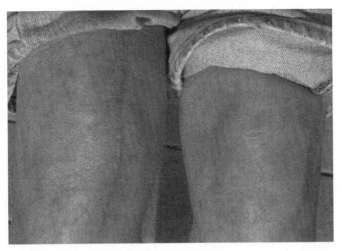

Have you been plagued with debilitating joint pain and inflammation? Do you wake up with stiff, aching joints? Do you feel sore every time you move? You are not alone. An estimated 46 million Americans suffer from the painful effects of arthritis.* Glucosamine helps prevent cartilage loss. Chondroitin rapidly regenerates new cartilage. Methylsulfonylmethane (MSM) reduces painful inflammation throughout the entire body.

Take Glucosamine, Chondroitin and MSM to treat and prevent arthritis. Cartilage is eighty-two percent water, so stay hydrated for your health! Always consult with your physician before stopping or starting any medication.

Barefoot Walking

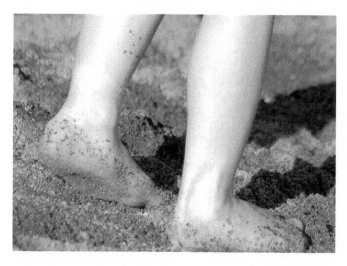

Barefoot walking builds strength of the small muscles inside of the arch of the foot, providing greater stability, balance and support.* The toes function better to grip the ground. Shoes actually can make our foot muscles weaker because shoes do not allow foot structures to move freely.

Try walking barefooted today at a soft surface such as carpet, sand or grass. How did you feel afterwards?

Power of Attitude

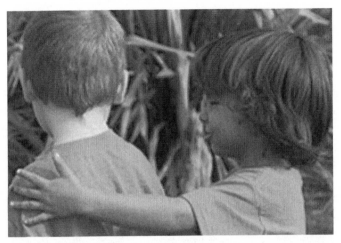

We've all heard the saying, "Treat every human being just the way that you would want to be treated." We all need an attitude adjustment about treating others. We need to treat others by who they are, not by what they do. This change of attitude will improve your wellbeing a great deal.

Treat everyone you meet today with same attitude of respect, love and grace. Treat those who don't usually get treated too well with more care and attention.

Life Saving Vitamin D

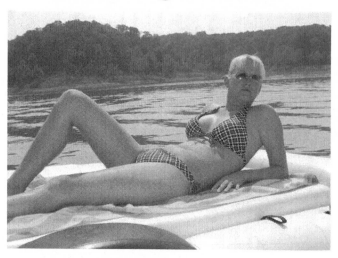

Vitamin D supports the immune system by increasing natural killer cells. It helps the body to process sugar more efficiently. Vitamin D also supports cardiovascular and colon health. It strengthens your muscles and reduces muscle pain. Lack of vitamin D is linked to seventeen different types of cancer.*

Have cod liver oil, salmon, sardines, tuna, egg yolk or beef liver to boost your vitamin D level. And of course, spend at least fifteen minutes each day in the sun to boost your Vitamin D levels.

Encourage Yourself

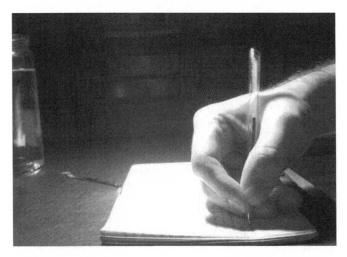

When you feel like nothing is going right, you're bored, depressed or overwhelmed, write down what you have accomplished so far in your life. Divide into categories such as family career, finances, spiritual or pleasure. By the time you finish creating the list, you will be encouraged about how much you have accomplished.

Encourage yourself daily with all your daily accomplishments. Read them aloud and tell yourself what you have done.

Strong and Energetic CoQ10

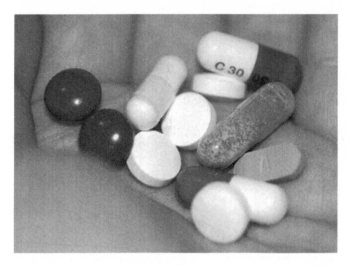

Coenzyme-Q10 is a powerful antioxidant that supports your entire cardiovascular system and protects against free-radical damage.* Plus, it's an outstanding natural energy producer that keeps your heart and body strong. It also supports normal blood pressure and blood lipid levels.

Meat and fish are high in CoQ10. In addition, sesame seeds, walnuts, soybeans, olive oil, parsley, broccoli, grapes, cauliflower and avocados are rich in CoQ10. CoQ10 is especially beneficial for anyone that has, or still does, smoke. Always consult with your physician before stopping or starting any medication.

Kind Words

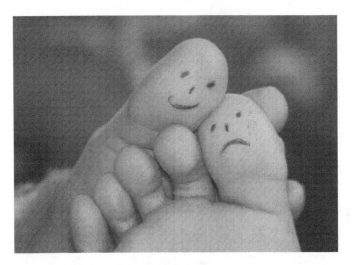

Kind words can be short and easy to speak, but their echoes are truly endless.

Speak only kind words to everyone you meet or talk to today. Notice how you feel at the end of the day.

Self Massage of Your Foot

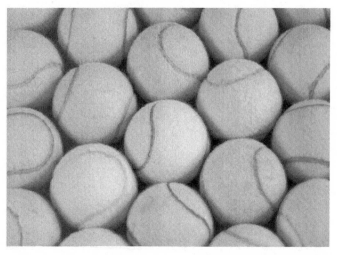

Foot massage therapy and deep friction massage work to increase blood flow, which will relax tight muscles and joints.* If you don't have massage therapy readily available, self massage by rolling the arch or your foot with a golf ball or tennis ball. If there is pain and inflammation in the bottom of the foot, use a frozen water bottle and roll the arch over the bottle.

Try the self massage of your foot today. Use different balls to create relieving effects.

Chromium Deficiency

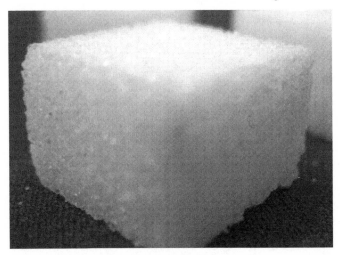

High consumption of refined sugar and grains causes deficiency in chromium.* Chromium is an essential trace mineral that enhances the body's sensitivity to insulin for sugar and fat metabolism as it facilitates insulin's uptake of glucose into the cells. The preferred form of chromium is chromium picolinate, and the recommended dosage for blood sugar support is 200 mcg daily, taken with meals.

If your sugar level is not well controlled, eat foods rich in chromium, such as potatoes, garlic, grapes, broccoli, whole grains, green beans, apples and bananas.

Easy Relief for Hot Flashes

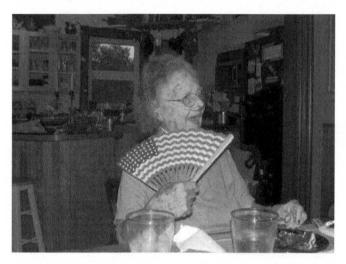

Research showed that menopausal women who added 20 grams of soy powder a day (about four tablespoons) to their diets reported significantly reduced their hot flashes and night sweats. Soy contains *isoflavones*, compounds that mimic the beneficial effects of estrogen without its risks. Estrogen-replacement therapy raises the risks of breast and ovarian cancer.*

Try soy if you have hot flashes and night sweats. Be careful not to buy genetically modified soy products, for it is dangerous to our health. If possible, get organic soy powder.

Great Service

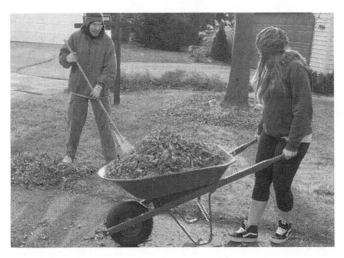

"Do all the good you can, by all the means you can, in all the ways you can, in all the places you can, at all the times you can, to all the people you can, as long as you ever can." - John Wesley

You can begin this service mentality by looking for small tasks that no one else wants to do. Start from your family and friends then expand from there.

Are You Tired and Cranky?

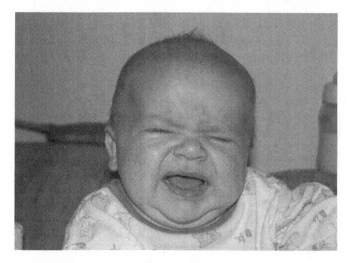

You may be deficient in iodine if you have fatigue and low energy, muscle aches, feeling depressed or irritable, cloudy thinking, memory lapses, constipation, dry skin, brittle fingernails, and overall weakness.* Iodine is a mineral that is an essential ingredient to make thyroid hormones, which control the body's entire metabolism.

Eat iodine rich food today to re-energize your body. Try haddock, cod, eggs, malt bread, sea kelp and seaweeds to boost your iodine and your health!

Good Digestion

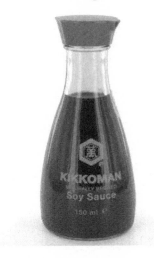

When you have gas, bloating, aches, pains, skin problems, lack of energy, weight gain and weak immunity, you may have poor digestion. The simplest, most effective way to re-energize your digestion and overall well being is to replenish the good bacteria in your intestines by adding probiotics to your diet.*

For your good digestion, take probiotic-rich foods such as sauerkraut, soy sauce, kimchi and organic yogurt. You can take a supplement with at least 10 billion probiotics in it.

Painful Blisters

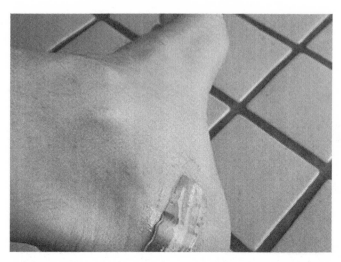

A blister is an accumulation of fluid just underneath the top layer of skin. Excessive friction, pressure, and moisture on the skin cause fluid to build up.* Avoidance is the key. Proper fitting socks and shoes are the most important factor. Protective padding is helpful to prevent recurrence of blisters.

If you have a blister, pop it with aseptic needle in the edge of the blister (not in the center) and apply antibiotic ointment and dressing. To avoid infection, do not take the cover off the blister until it is healed.

Have You Been Procrastinating Lately?

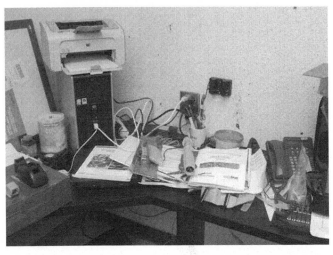

Have you been feeling lazy? Are you indecisive? Do you always wait for the "perfect" moment? Do you not do something unless it is convenient for you? Are you afraid of getting started on something that you may not finish? Do you find yourself looking for reasons that something will not work out? If you do, you may be procrastinating now.

The next time you find yourself procrastinating, stop and ask yourself why. Then pick a task that you have been procrastinating and just start on it. It is always helpful to start on something easy for you first.

You May Have Food Allergies

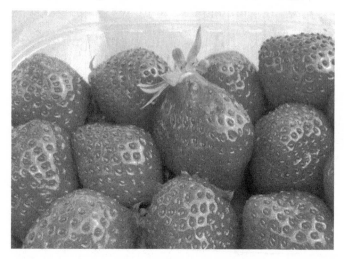

If you regularly experience allergic reactions such as eczema, hives, hay fever, asthma attacks, diarrhea and plain not feeling good, you may have a food allergy to one of the many common allergenic foods: dairy products, soy, eggs, peanuts, wheat, shellfish, corn and strawberries. Most of us are at least mildly allergic to synthetic colors and chemical additives found in packaged and canned goods.*

If you have the above allergy symptoms, quit all the common allergen foods for three weeks. Then, reintroduce one food at a time slowly back into your diet. You will notice the allergy causing food right away.

Contentment

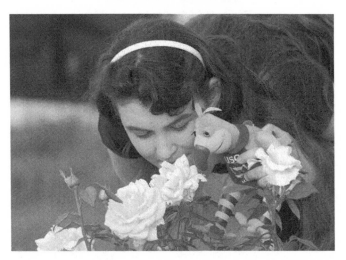

Contentment does not dependent upon circumstances. Contentment is something one has to learn. Most of us are naturally discontent because we compare. We compare houses, cars, income, clothes, looks, talents, skills and even where we go on vacations. We will never be content if we always want more.

Be content today with what you have and stop comparing. Happiness isn't dependent on how much or how little we have.

How to Beat
Arthritis Naturally

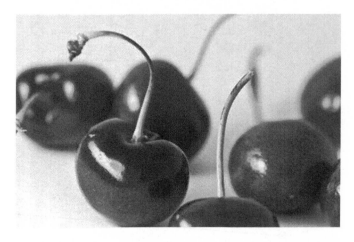

16 million Americans suffer from osteoarthritis.*
You can beat this arthritis with 1.5gms of glucosamine, 1.2gms of chondroitin, 5,000IU of
Vitamin A, 4gms of Vitamin C, 400IU of Vitamin
E, 200mcgms of Selenium and Bioflavonoids
such as green tea, berries, onions, garlic, citrus
fruits, cherries and plums.

Instead of reaching for aspirin, ibuprofen or
other nonsteroidal anti-inflammatory drugs
(NSAIDs) to control arthritis pain, try the above
natural ingredients today.

Dr. S. Don Kim

More Veggies for Kids

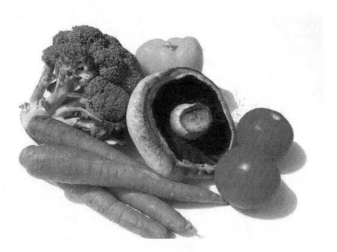

Kids will eat more vegetables when healthful produce is part of their main meals instead of side dishes. Add pureed cooked vegetables to ground-meat dishes like meatloaf and hamburgers. Substitute shredded carrots, chopped spinach or zucchini for ground meat in lasagna or a casserole. Add pureed or shredded vegetables to homemade muffins, cookies, cakes and breads.*

Make sure your children get enough vegetables every day. Be creative with your recipes to integrate more veggies for your kids' wellbeing.

Itchy Athlete's Foot

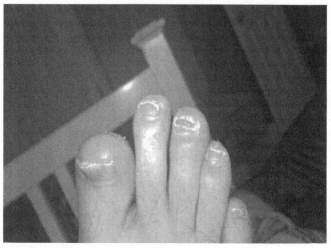

Athlete's foot is a skin infection caused by fungus which thrives in a dark, moist, warm environment such as a shoe. It thrives in damp areas such as swimming pools, showers, and locker rooms. We sweat twenty times more on our palms and soles than other parts of body, fungus loves to stay on our feet. Athlete's foot produces itchy, dry, scaling skin. It is commonly seen on the soles of the feet and in between the toes.*

Keep your feet as dry as possible after a sporting event or shower. If your feet sweat a lot, you may need to change your socks and shoes during the day. Use anti-fungal powders in the shoes while not being used and do not wear the same shoes two days in a row.

Dr. S. Don Kim

Everything is a Miracle

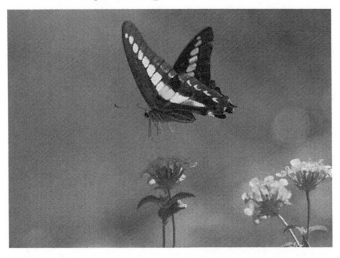

"There are only two ways to live your life. One is as though nothing is a miracle. The other is as though everything is a miracle." - Albert Einstein

Your heart pumps almost 100,000 times a day without your input; your eyes can distinguish 10 million different colors; your nose can smell 10,000 different odors and your red blood cells are replenishing 2.4 million cells every second. You are a true miracle!

Ease the Jet Lag

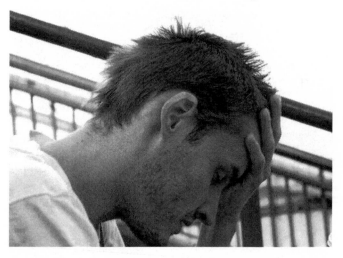

When you fly across several time zones, you disrupt the body's circadian rhythms. The condition of jet lag may last many days, and recovery rates of 1 day per eastward time zone or 1 day per 1.5 westward time zones. Symptoms are headaches, fatigue, insomnia, constipation, diarrhea and mild depression.*

To ease jet lag, you should avoid drinking alcohol during flight, limit caffeine, drink plenty of water and take melatonin 0.3 to 0.5mg.

Leafy Folic Acid

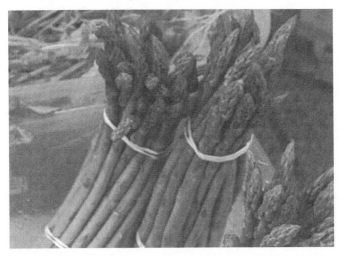

Folic acid (vitamin B9) is known to be essential for pregnant women to prevent birth defects of a child. In addition, folic acid is necessary to synthesize and repair DNA, produce healthy red blood cells and prevent anemia.* The word folic acid comes from the Latin word "folium" which actually means "leaf".

Eat folic acid rich foods today, such as leafy green vegetables (spinach, asparagus, turnip greens), legumes (beans, peas, lentils), baker's yeast, sunflower seeds and fruits (oranges, pine-apples, cantaloupe, honey dew and grapefruit).

Be an Optimist

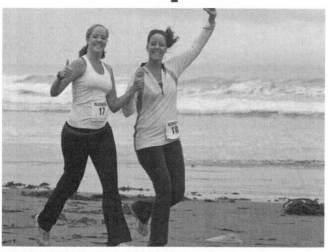

"A pessimist sees the difficulty in every opportunity; an optimist sees the opportunity in every difficulty." -Winston Churchill

Are you going through a difficult time right now? What is the opportunity in that? Talk to a family member or a friend about this and see the situation as an optimist.

Scrape Your Tongue

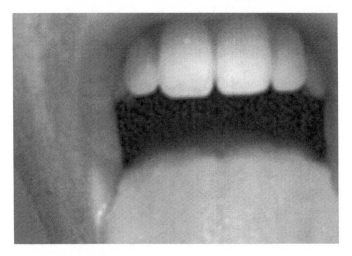

Every day, infectious bacteria, viruses, fungus and yeast along with food particles and cellular debris collect on the rough surface on the back of the tongue. This can cause tooth decay, gum disease, sore throats and colds as well as bad breath.*

Clean the top of your tongue twice a day with a scraping device after breakfast and before bedtime to prevent bad breath and infections in and around your mouth today.

Painful Sacs on Your Feet

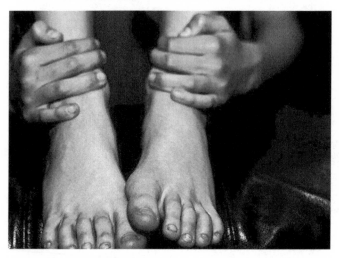

Bursitis is an inflammation of a small fluid-filled sac, called a bursa, located near a joint, bone or tendon. The bursa, which protects the area from friction, can become inflamed from repetitive motion or irritation from shoes. In the foot, the back of the heel and the top of the toes are most often affected. These sacs cause localized redness, swelling and pain.*

Make sure your shoes are not rubbing these areas to cause irritation. Treatment may include local ice therapy, non-steroidal anti-inflammatory drugs (NSAIDs), such as ibuprofen, padding around the sacs to avoid irritation, or corticosteroid injections to help reduce inflammation and relieve pain.

Hope

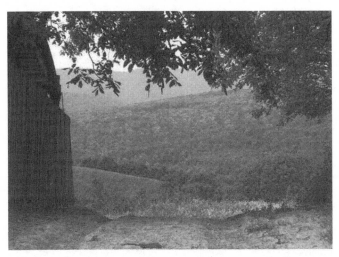

Hope did not exist in the beginning. Just like a road that did not exist. It came to exist when people walked one by one creating the road. Hope starts from nothing. Hope exists for those who believe in it. It does not exist for those who don't believe.*

Let's hope for better health. Believe that you and your loved ones have the power to improve their health no matter how sick they are right now.

Give Generously and Cheerfully

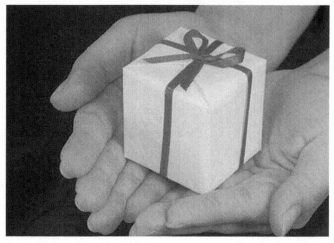

Remember this: whoever sows sparingly will also reap sparingly. And whoever sows generously will also reap generously. Each one should give what he has decided in his heart to give, not reluctantly or under compulsion for God loves a cheerful giver. (2 Corinthians 9:6-7)

Practice the virtue of giving today. Remember whatever you give, it will be given unto you.

Dr. S. Don Kim

What Causes Migraines

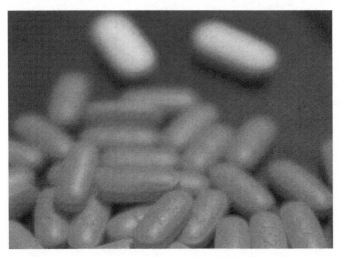

Migraines affect 18% of women and 6% of men in America.* Migraines are not just any headache. They are severe throbbing pain that can keep you home from work, disrupt your family life and leave you significantly disabled. Alcohol (beer and red wine), irregular meals, irregular sleep pattern, Aspartame (NutraSweet), MSG, nitrates in processed meats, tyramine in cheeses, baked bread, chopped liver, perfume, caffeine and gluten in grains can cause migraines.

If you have migraines, you should avoid the above foods or behaviors. Check to make sure you are not allergic to any of the substances above or other artificial ingredients.

Use it or Lose it

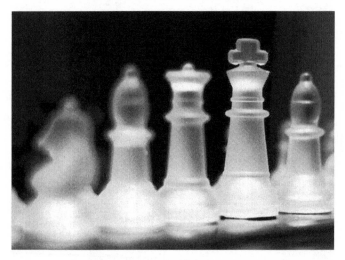

The longer you neglect your talents or special skills that you developed over the years, the harder it is to restore them and the less likely you will be able to bring them back to their old levels of excellence. The deterioration of our abilities occurs due to disuse of both mental and physical abilities.

Your physical and mental health depends on your skills. Practice your old skills such as tennis or chess to sharpen your abilities today. Let's bring them back to life.

Cold Feet?

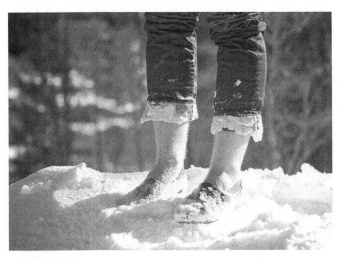

Cold feet are commonly a result of medical conditions that cause poor blood flow in the legs or feet, Raynaud's phenomenon (cold sensitivity which causes a spasm of the blood vessels), and heart disease. Other causes of cold feet include hormonal abnormalities such as hypothyroidism and adrenal insufficiency, nerve disorders such as peripheral neuropathy and fibromyalgia, and autoimmune disorders (lupus, scleroderma).

Keep your feet warm by soaking in warm Epsom salt water daily. Try a hot pack behind your knees to increase blood flow to the toes. Quit smoking and caffeine. Ginkgo biloba leaves and fish oil supplements have shown to improve cold feet.*

Open Your Windows

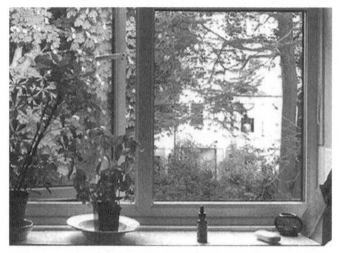

Did you know that indoors could be up to five times more polluted than outdoors? 80% of indoor pollution is from our own skin shedding. Every 25-45 days you have a completely new skin layer on your entire body. You are shedding an average of forty pounds of skin in your life-time, loaded with bacteria, fungus and dust mites in it! * You need to open your windows daily to get fresh air and reduce indoor pollution.

Open your windows today to get fresh air. Make it a habit to do this as often as you can especially in the winter, when we spend more time inside. Air conditioning is not enough to clean the air inside; you need to let fresh air in daily!

Be That Friend

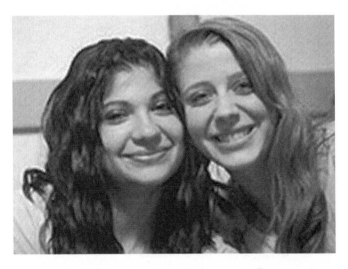

You should have a friend who you can call on when you feel down or depressed. This friend should lift your spirit back up to be happy again by making you laugh and be encouraged. We are all so lucky to have a few friends like this to call on. Take time to cultivate this type of friendship with others. Your life will be enriched.

Also, you can be that friend who people call on when they feel down and depressed. When you are that friend, you will more likely attract this type of relationship for when you need it.

Natural Air Filters

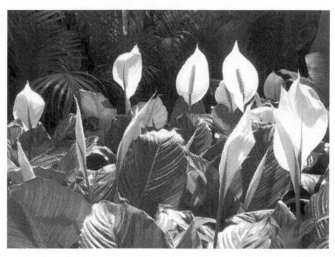

Did you know that houseplants such as aloe, Chinese evergreen, English ivy, ficus, golden pothos, corn plants, peace lily, spider plants and elephant earphilodendron can serve as natural air filters? It's true! Plants can remove indoor air pollutants such as formaldehyde and carbon monoxide.*

Grow a houseplant to decrease indoor pollution. You will enjoy their beauty as well.

Dr. S. Don Kim

Are You Getting Enough Magnesium?

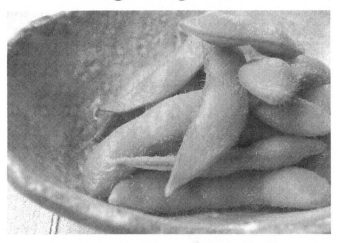

Up to 70% of women are magnesium deficient. Women taking calcium to fight osteoporosis should take enough magnesium too because the body aims to keep the two minerals in balance. Without enough magnesium, calcium is simply excreted and not absorbed.*

If you are already taking enough calcium supplements, you should add 200mg of Magnesium. You can add magnesium rich foods like green leafy vegetables, whole-grain breads, soybeans, tofu, organic milk or yogurt.

Is Your Athletic Child Limping?

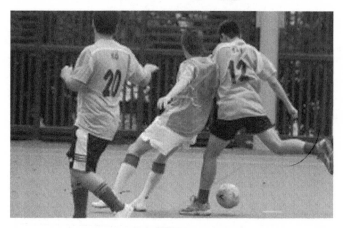

If your child is limping after playing soccer, track or basketball, he or she may have a calcaneal apophysitis or Sever's disease. Repetitive stress to the growth plate of the heel bone between the ages of eight and fourteen causes pain and swelling of the heel. Your child may have pain in the back or bottom of the heel, limp, walk on their toes or have difficulty running, jumping or participating in usual activities or sports.*

Rest from all the sports activities including gym class until the pain improves. Immobilizing in a boot or cast will help recovery. Heel lifts inserted into shoes to take tension off of the calf muscles and tendons are helpful. Physical therapy also promotes healing.

Yes I Can!

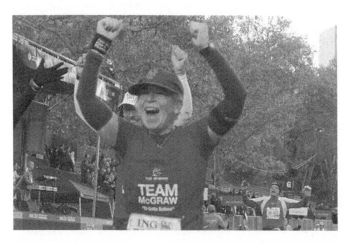

"Nothing can stop the man with the right mental attitude from achieving his goal; nothing on earth can help a man with the wrong mental attitude."
-Thomas Jefferson

If you have a difficult time getting the right mental attitude, just say "Yes, I can!" and repeat this mantra to yourself all day long. You may be surprised at the result.

Sound Asleep

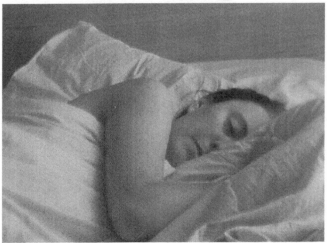

50-70% of Americans suffer from insufficient nightly rest. More than 42 million sleeping pills are prescribed each year. Also over $100 billion is lost because oflack of sleep through lost productivity, medical expenses and sick leave. Research shows that Baroque style classical music fights insomnia very effectively.*

Use Baroque music before you go to sleep. You will realize such calmness with this type of music. You can also use this music during your relaxation time too.

Asthma Proof Your Home

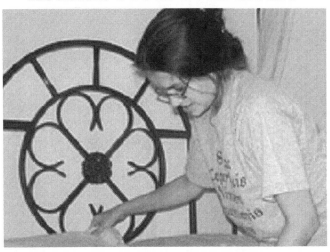

Nearly 20 million Americans have asthma. You need to asthma proof your home to fight this disease.* Remove all carpeting. Encase your mattress, box spring and pillows in airtight vinyl covers. Eliminate water leaks to decrease humidity. Dust frequently with special cloths that prevent dust from scattering. Purchase salt lamps to create negative ions in each room of the house.

Create an asthma proof home today, especially if you or your loved ones suffer from this disease.

Character

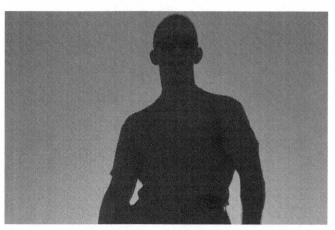

"Character cannot be developed in ease and quiet. Only through experiences of trial and suffering can the soul be strengthened, vision cleared, ambition inspired and success achieved."
- Helen Keller

Think of those experiences that have shaped your character in the past and the ones that are shaping it now. Remember that there is a reason for everything and none of your experiences will be wasted.

Shoe Contact Dermatitis

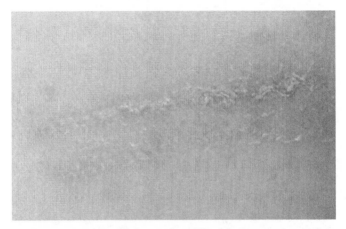

On average, American families buy seven pairs of shoes annually. Shoes are made with leather, rubber and other synthetic materials. In addition, cements and dichromates are used in tanning; dyes, rubber additives, anti-mildew agents, formaldehyde, nickel eyelets and nickel arch supports are added during the manufacturing process. These materials can cause contact dermatitis of the foot with redness, itchiness, and small blisters, usually occurring within 24 to 72 hours of exposure to the irritant.*

Try moist compresses and cool moist soaks for five to ten minutes first, followed by air-drying. Then try moisturizing cream with glycerin and alpha-hydroxy acids. If they don't work, you need topical corticosteroid prescribed by your foot doctor.

Red Meat and Non-Hodgkin's Lymphoma

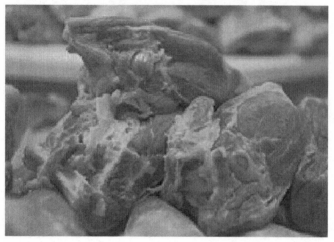

Eating red meat increases the risk of developing non-Hodgkin's Lymphoma, a white blood cell cancer. A study of more than 35,000 women showed that those who ate the most red meat were almost twice as likely to develop this cancer. In addition, those who ate the most animal fat also had 1 ½ times the risk of developing the cancer as those who ate the least.*

If you are concerned about this type of cancer, cut down on the consumption of meat, especially red meat. If you want to have meat products, stay with free range, organic meats to avoid many toxins, such as hormones and antibiotics.

Tomatoes for Prostate Cancer

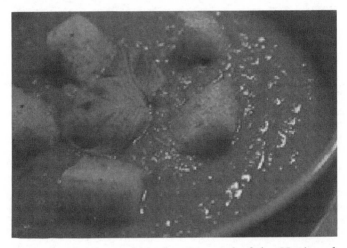

A study conducted by the Journal of the National Cancer Institute showed that almost 50,000 men who ate two or more servings of cooked tomatoes each week reduced the risk of prostate cancer by 30%.* When they ate 10 or more servings each week, the risk dropped to 50%. This is from the high content of Lycopene, an antioxidant in tomatoes. Cooked tomatoes seemed to bring out more lycopene than raw ones.

Eat cooked tomatoes today to fight prostate cancer. Try other cancer fighting foods such as broccoli, cabbage, soybeans and carrots too.

Stand Tall

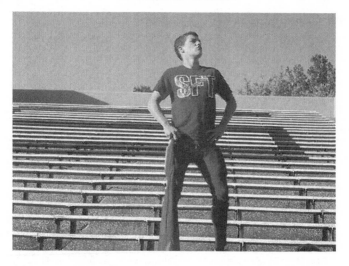

By maintaining good posture, you will look 10 pounds thinner and 10 years younger.* Stand tall and breathe from below your navel. You will notice your chest upward, stomach flatter and torso longer and thinner.

Practice this posture in front of mirror. Remember this posture whenever you see yourself hunched over after sitting for awhile. You won't have that old, tired and hunched look any longer.

Manage Your Thoughts

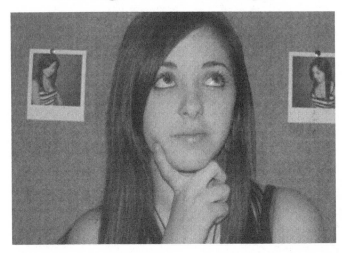

When you focus your thoughts on what you want rather than what you don't want, you will feel more powerful. Your thoughts determine your actions. Before the action takes place, they determine your direction. Your life will flow toward a weak direction if you think of weak thoughts and toward a strong direction with strong thoughts. Therefore, you need to manage your thoughts, which will manage your character and eventually your whole life.

Focus on thoughts that will make you strong and powerful today. Let's focus on what you want in your life rather than what you don't want in life.

How to Cure Bad Smell on Your Feet

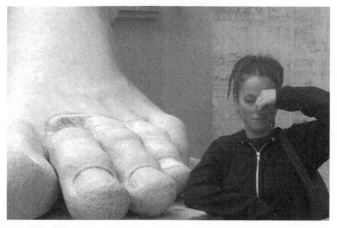

Foot odor is produced by bacteria and/or fungus that grows in the shoes and attaches to the skin. Some bacteria can actually eat away the top layer of the skin, producing a foul odor. Hair on your feet, especially on your toes, may contribute to the odor's intensity by adding surface area in which bacteria can thrive. Some synthetic materials used in shoes, when mixed with sweat and bacteria, can produce smelly feet.

Use four pinches of baking soda (sodium bicarbonate) daily to eliminate the odor. Use two pinches inside the sock and two on the insole of the shoe. Try soaking your feet in a tub of iced tea. Use zinc and castor oil cream on the feet to reduce odor.*

Dr. S. Don Kim

Colorful Fruits and Vegetables for Cataracts

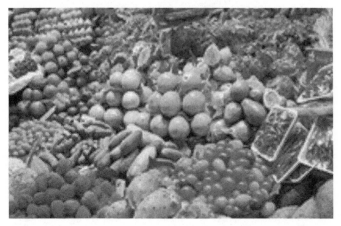

A cataract is a clouding of the lens of the eye, which is responsible for 48% of blindness, affecting about 18 million people worldwide. Much of the damage is caused by UV light, exposure to radiation and secondary effects of diseases such as diabetes, hypertension and advanced age.* These are all results of free radical damage from oxidation, which is essentially the aging process.

Try consuming rich antioxidants to reverse this damage on the eyes. Brightly colored fruits and vegetables, especially squash, spinach, broccoli, oranges, carrots and sweet potatoes are helpful for this condition. They are rich in vitamin A and C as well as beta-carotene.

Grape Juice for Blood Clots

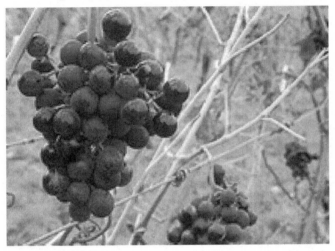

The Journal of the American College of Cardiology published a study that purple grape juice prevents dangerous blood clots more effectively than aspirin. These purple grapes have flavonoids that reduce clotting of platelets by about 40%. The similar effect can be achieved with red wine.*

Enjoy a glass of red wine or 100% fresh grape juice to reduce clotting of blood. Remember, aspirin can cause many side effects. The most common is internal bleeding.

Ballroom Dance

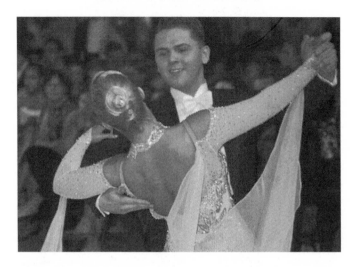

Ballroom dancing is a set of partner dances, which are enjoyed both socially and competitively around the world. They are dances like the Waltz, Tango, Foxtrot, Cha Cha, Rumba, Swing and Mambo. It is an excellent alternative for those who have a hard time exercising but love to dance. This helps you develop coordination, balance, rhythm, strength and flexibility.*

Look for a ballroom dance studio nearby. This is one of the best therapies for married couples both physically and mentally. Your intimacy will be enhanced.

Watch Out for Liquid Supplements

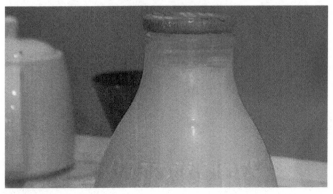

Many liquid supplements such as Ensure, Boost, Resource and Sustacal are being promoted as meal replacements. These liquid supplements contain water, soy, milk protein, sugar, oil, and artificial vitamins and minerals. They lack natural nutrients and fiber that we need on a daily basis. They are not a substitute for real food.*

Avoid these liquid supplements as meal replacements. If you have elderly parents or family members, advise them to eat more fruits and vegetables. Use protein shakes or vegetable juices in place of these liquid supplements.

Pump Bump

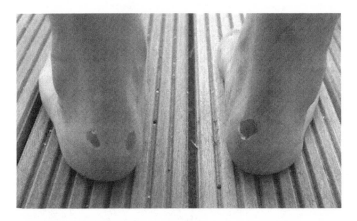

Haglund's Deformity is a bony enlargement on the back of the heel. The soft tissue near the Achilles tendon becomes irritated when the bony enlargement rubs against shoes. This deformity is often called "pump bump" because the rigid backs of women's pump-style shoes can create pressure that aggravates the enlargement when walking. In fact, any shoes with a rigid back, such as ice skates, men's dress shoes, or women's pumps, can cause this irritation.*

Stretching exercises help relieve tension from the Achilles tendon. Heel lifts placed inside the shoe decrease the pressure on the heel. Physical therapymodalities, such as ultrasound, electro-stimulation and deep tissue massage can help to reduce inflammation. Surgery may be necessary if none of the treatments above are effective.

Good Company

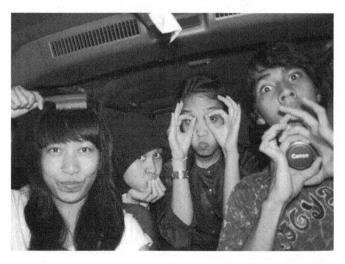

"Associate with men of good quality if you esteem your own reputation, for it is better to be alone than in bad company."-George Washington

Have good people around you who will make you feel great all the time and you will become that person who they call on when they want to feel good. Then you will attract more of those good people in your life.

Dr. S. Don Kim

How to Reduce Stress at Work

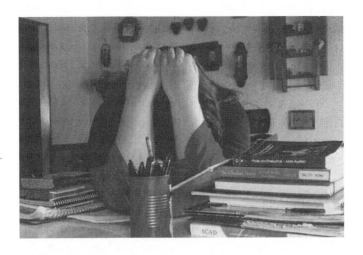

Your career can demand high psychological stress without control, discretion over tasks, or autonomy.

Take three deep breaths every half an hour to release tension. Get up from your chair after the breaths and look outside a window to briefly relieve your eyes and mind from your tasks. Set aside an hour or two each morning, preferably without taking phone calls, and perform the most difficult tasks during this uninterrupted, most productive time of the day.

Watch out for Dangerous Diets

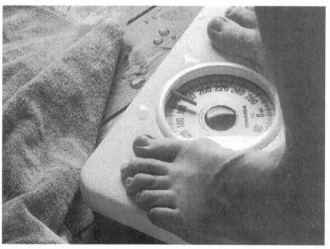

Watch out for these dangerous diet claims: loss of more than two to three pounds per week, restricting large quantities of specific foods, do not emphasize lifestyle changes or exercise programs, promote miracle foods or supplements, or do not show time tested and scientifically researched strategies to keep the weight maintained after the loss.

Remember keeping the weight off is more difficult than losing the weight. If you lose weight slowly and healthfully with lifestyle changes and exercise, you will be able to maintain it for a long time.*

Have a Soul Mate

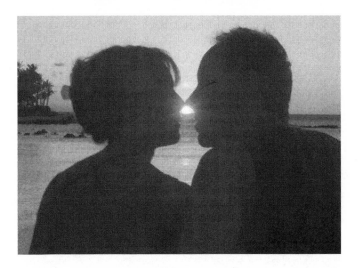

Up to age 70, marriage reduces the risk of premature death and disability about 50%. Having a friend, lover or companion to share your life and feelings is one of the most important health insurance policies you can have.*

Spend time to nurture a soul mate or a friend. Owning a pet also enables you to interact emotionally with them.

Be Careful with Toning Shoes

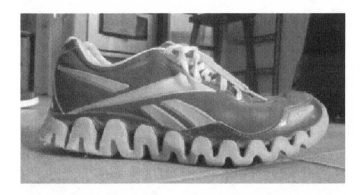

Researchers from the American Council on Exercise put the popular toning shoes to the test.*
They recruited people to wear EasyTones, Shapeups and MBTs and walk on treadmills. When the researchers measured the muscle activities, they found no significant increase in muscle activities comparing toning shoes to normal sneakers. In addition, toning shoes can cause tendonitis, especially in the tendo-achilles and other tendons supporting the foot and ankle.

The only time the toner shoes are helpful is when you have arthritis of foot or ankle. They allow rocking motion of the foot to lessen the pressure to the arthritic joints. If you want to wear the toning shoes, be careful not to fall and to slowly get used to the shoes.

How to Prevent Dry Skin

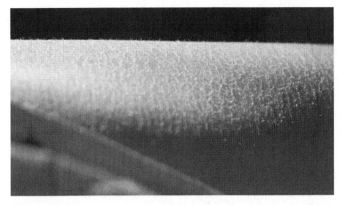

Dry skin is the number one cause of skin irritation and itchiness. Dry skin happens more often in the winter when the cold air outside and the hot air inside creates low humidity. This causes the skin to lose moisture and it may crack and peel. Bathing too long or hand washing too frequently, especially if one is using harsh soaps, may also contribute to dry skin. Dry skin can also be caused by a deficiency of water, vitamin A, vitamin D, and enough proper salt in the diet.*

Nourish your skin by hydrating adequately every day. Eat a healthy diet of mostly raw fruits and vegetables and increase omega-3 fatty acids by consuming flax seed or fish. Use only mineral salts and bathe with salts to help dry skin slough off. Use organic moisturizers such as pure coconut oil.

Go Up Side Down

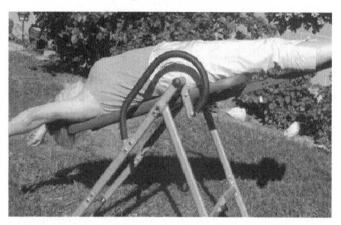

Hanging upside down (Inversion Therapy) has been used to help back and neck pain for over 2500 years, since Hippocrates. We fight gravity daily, and average person loses ½ to 2 inches of height as they reach our senior years. Inversion therapy is a powerful way to improve circulation, relieve stress, heighten mental alertness, increase flexibility, improve posture and realign your back, neck and spine.*

Try inversion therapy today especially if you have neck or back pain. Make sure you start at only 1-2 minutes a day, increasing angle and duration slowly. Be cautious if you have hypertension, osteoporosis, heart problems, hernia, spinal implants or have recently had surgery. Please consult your physician before you start this therapy.

Enjoy Sweet Potatoes

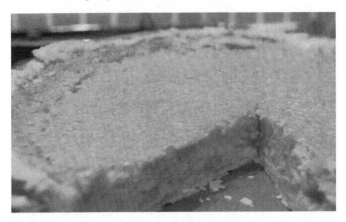

Sweet potatoes are tasty and highly nutritious root vegetables. They are high in beta-carotene, vitamins B1, B6, niacin, C, E, as well as calcium, iron, and potassium. The nutritive content is great for maintaining regular bowel health, healthy skin, and relief from asthma and arthritis. Adding sweet potatoes to your diet may reverse anemia and high blood pressure and they may contribute to preventing heart disease, strokes, and several types of cancers and may even remove heavy metals such as mercury, lead, cadmium and copper from the body.*

Look for firm, smooth skinned sweet potatoes. The brighter and darker the color, the more beta carotene it contains. They can be enjoyed raw, grated into salads, pureed, or baked and cooked into pies, puddings, and soups.

Potassium and Blood Pressure

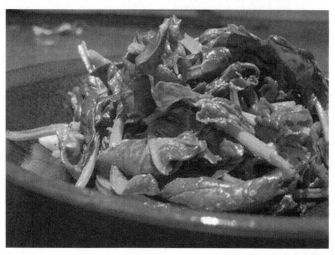

An increased intake of potassium can lower blood pressure even more so than lowering your sodium level. To keep the blood pressure under control, you should take five times more potassium than sodium.* Unfortunately, most Americans eat two times more sodium than potassium, due to the prevalence of high sodium-processed foods. It is important to keep your salt consumption under control, but it is more important to increase potassium consumption.

Add potassium rich foods to your diet, such as avocado, mushrooms, broccoli, brussels sprouts, and spinach. Keep the salt consumption under control and use only mineral salts.

Dangerous Barefoot Running

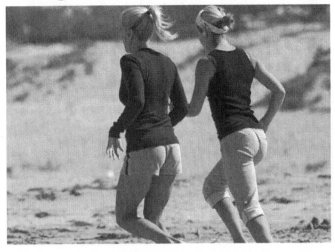

Lately, barefoot running became more popular with promises of fewer injuries while running. Running is a very individual thing--varying from person to person--and you should experiment cautiously to see if barefoot running works for you. Barefoot running can reduce the pressure to the knee up to 38%.* On the other hand, it can cause metatarsal (ball of the foot) fractures, capsulitis and bursitis of joints of the ball of the foot.

Check to make sure your feet are able to handle barefoot running first before you embark on your journey. If you have a pronated type of foot, you should avoid barefoot running.

Look Beyond Your Obstacles

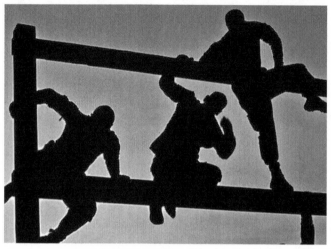

Do you have a little voice in your head telling you that you will not succeed? Do you feel constantly distracted by people or things around you? Do you often attempt to take shortcuts? Are you impatient about discouraging delays? These are the obstacles you face when you try to achieve your goals in life.

Look beyond these obstacles and see the joy of achieving your goals. If you can see the goals as the bigger picture, your obstacles will become smaller in comparison. When you view your challenges as larger, your joy and chances of achieving your goals will not be as easy.

Watercress Fights Cancer

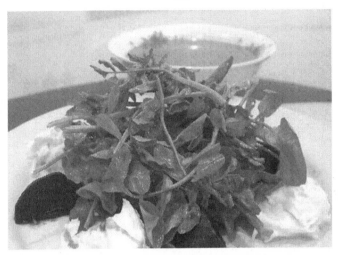

Watercress is a peppery and sweet tasting green leafy vegetable. This member of the cabbage family contains significant amounts of iron, calcium and folic acid, in addition to vitamins A and C. It also appears to have cancer-suppressing properties, particularly effective in preventing colon, lung and breast cancer. Its high iodine content makes watercress have a strengthening effect on the thyroid gland, beneficial for sufferers of hypothyroidism.*

Add fresh watercress to your salad, soup or sandwich. Enjoy this wonderful health food as many places as you can, especially if you suffer from cancer or thyroid problems.

Overeating and Heartburn

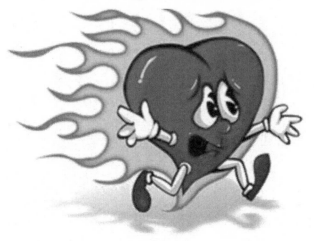

A Japanese proverb says, "If you only eat to 70% of stomach's capacity, you won't need a doctor." Overeating is the primary cause of heartburn.* Heartburn--also known as acid reflux--occurs when stomach acid flows back up into the esophagus. Because the esophagus has no protective lining, the acid can cause pain, coughing, and asthma-like symptoms. If you feel too stuffed and sleepy after your meal, you overate.

Look down at your plate. If the amount of food on your plate is bigger than your two palms, you are overeating. Portion control is essential to your health.

Boosting Self Esteem

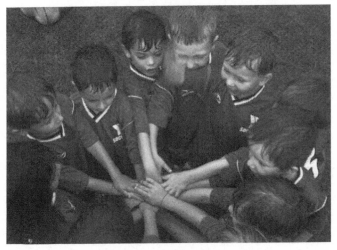

"Outstanding leaders go out of their way to boost the self-esteem of their personnel. If people believe in themselves, it's amazing what they can accomplish. " - Sam Walton, founder of Wal-Mart.

Tell someone how great he or she is. Tell yourself how great you are. Let's believe in ourselves by boosting our self-esteem. We definitely can use it.

Dangerous High Heels

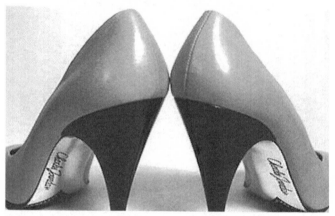

When you switch from a one-inch heel to a three-inch heel, you put seven times the amount of pressure on the ball of your foot.* Women's foot pain often comes from wearing these dangerous shoes. They offer less support and more crowding within the toe box, which can lead to hammertoes, bunions, blisters, tendonitis, ankle sprains, ingrown toenails, and neuromas.

Use high heels sparingly. Try opting for roomier and more supportive shoes, and always have a more comfortable pair of shoes at work and home.

Dr. S. Don Kim

Stay Slim with Stevia

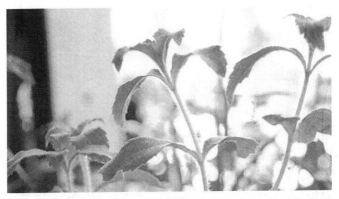

Stevia may be one of the most important refined sugar replacements ever discovered. It is an herb and shrub in the Chrysanthemum family native to South America. Stevia is thirty times sweeter than sugar in its unprocessed form, and when purified, it can be 250-300 times sweeter than sugar! It has zero calories, and is safe for diabetics.* Stevia users have reported reduced appetite and a reduction of their craving for sweets and fatty foods, making it a very effective addition to your diet. It also helps manage blood pressure.

Add stevia to your diet wherever you'd add sugar; it is excellent in cooking and baking. You can also use water-based stevia to any beverage. There are a number of stevia-sweetened products now making their way into mainstream markets.

Juice Your Celery

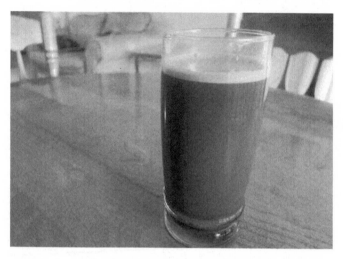

Celery is loaded with potassium and magnesium. Celery is also a good source of fiber and vitamins A, C, and E. Celery combats hypertension because it contains coumarin, a compound that relaxes the smooth muscle cells in the arterial walls, allowing the arteries to dilate and effectively lowering blood pressure.* Its cooling and calming properties make it an excellent addition to the diet for high-stress types and athletes. In addition, celery is a low-calorie food. Each eight-inch rib has only six calories, making it a healthy and replenishing snack.

Juice celery sticks in the morning. Celery is great raw, and it is also delicious cooked in soups, stews and casseroles.

Make a Difference

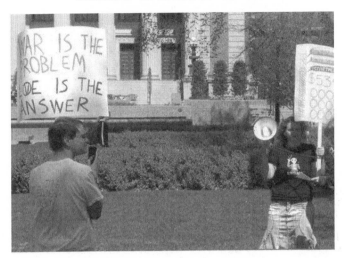

What is bothering you about the health of the world today? What concerns you about American family life? What annoys you about the school system? Do you think about certain social issues? Do you ponder the toxic elements of the environment we live in? Do you feel anxious about the unpredictable economic turmoil?

Make a list of the needs you see that seriously disturb you. Write down the ways you can use your gifts and talents to make a difference. Act now!

Soft Drinks Soften Bones

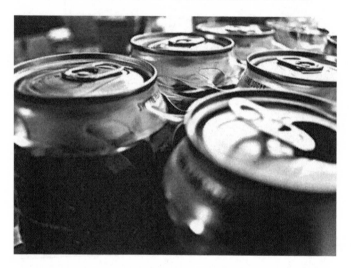

Americans drink 13.15 billion gallons of soft drinks every year.* The United States ranks first among countries for soft drink consumption. Each person drinks about 15 ounces a day -- a little more than one can. One of soda's major ingredients, phosphoric acid, has been linked to lower bone density in epidemiological studies. Phosphoric acid interferes with your body's ability to use calcium. This leads to softening of teeth and bones.

Reduce consumption of soft drinks or eliminate them completely for your bone health. Use water as your only source of fluid.

Fructose in Soda and Gout

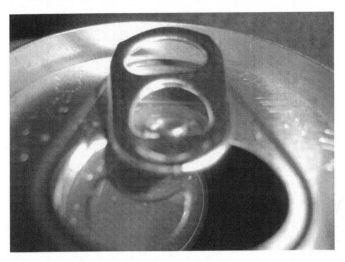

Gout affects an estimated two to five million Americans and it accounts for about 5% of all cases of arthritis. This painful form of arthritis targets big toe of your foot most commonly, then ankle, knee and spine in that order. Studies have shown an alarming trend between the increase in gout cases and the consumption of high levels of fructose. Sodas have high levels of fructose anywhere from 58% to 65% in the more popular brands.

If you or your loved ones have gout, you need to stay away from soda. So instead of grabbing that quick soda, grab your water bottle and you're ready to go!*

Sick Building Syndrome

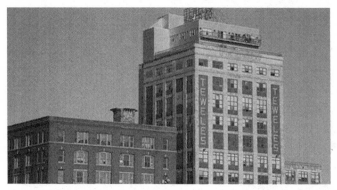

If you have watery eyes, runny nose, headaches, dizziness, nausea and a tightening sensation in the chest and these symptoms get worse while in the work environment but significantly improve during vacations or weekends, you may suffer from sick building syndrome. Modern office buildings can be the cause. They are built with toxic chemicals and built tight as a drum with poor ventilation, leaving allergens and irritants such as dander, molds, and dust mites with no place to go. These may be the cause of those symptoms.

Buy plants like a Dwarf date palm, Bamboo palm or Janet Craig to cleanse the air.* Keep your work area free of clutter, dust regularly and use a HEPA-type table top air purifier or salt lamp. See a nutritionist to detoxify your body every seasonal change. This is highly recommended especially if you have the above symptoms.

Avoid Flu Shots

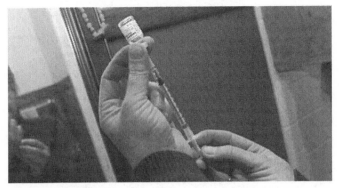

The flu shot contains thimerosal, a preservative made of mercury, one of the most toxic substances. The shot also contains other dangerous elements: a mixture of rotten egg proteins*, polysorbate 80, a potential carcinogen associated with infertility in animals; formaldehyde, a known carcinogen and Triton X-100, a detergent.

Avoid the flu in more healthful way: Hydrate daily with eight glasses of spring water and eat more fresh fruits and vegetables. Take 25,000-100,000 units of vitamin A, five to six grams of vitamin C, and 6,000-10,000 units of vitamin D daily. Take 10 billion probiotics. Flush your nose and gargle with organic salt water daily.

Quinoa, a Great Alternative to Rice and Pasta

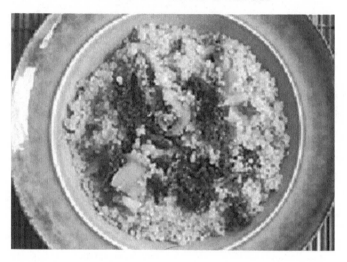

Quinoa looks like a grain, but it's a seed of a leafy green plant native to South America. It is rich in protein, fiber, magnesium and potassium. Quinoa has a low glycemic index and is an excellent alternative to starchy grains and pasta.* It is also wonderful for those who have gluten allergy.

Try Quinoa as a substitute for rice, pasta, or potatoes. You can use it for stuffing too. You can purchase it at local health food store.

Dr. S. Don Kim

Vitamin B12 Prevents Alzheimer's Disease

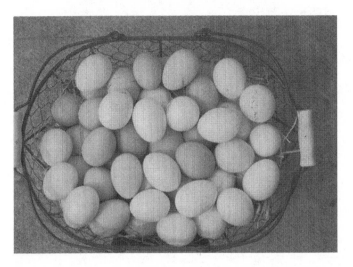

According to the Alzheimer's Disease Facts and Figures report for 2009, 5.3 million people in the U.S. have this disease and it's the sixth leading cause of death in the country. In the next 20 years Alzheimer's could affect as many as one in four Americans, more widespread than obesity and diabetes.* Vitamin B12 has been shown to be a benefit for memory stability, which helps the fight against Alzheimer's Disease.

Eat more Vitamin B12 rich foods such as chicken, eggs, fish, avocados, nuts, corn or oat meal, and soy. If you are a vegan, it is recommended that you take Vitamin B12 supplements.

Are Your Kids Wearing the Wrong Shoe Size?

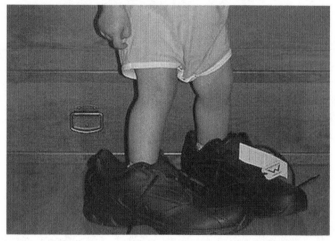

According to new research, four million children are wearing the wrong shoe size. The risks of children's shoes not fitting correctly are: blisters, pressure sores, and ingrown toenails for short-term problems. There should be no more than a 14mm gap between the big toe and end of a shoe in a new pair. Anything less than 8mm and it's time to get another pair.*

When you go shopping for new shoes, check the gap between the big toe and end of a shoe. If your child is going through a growth spurt, check the fitting more often.

Dr. S. Don Kim

Beat a Cold with Hydrogen Peroxide

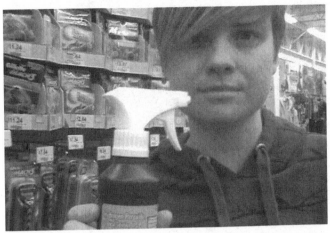

Each year about one billion colds affect the lives of Americans making it the most common infectious disease in the U.S. The biggest misconception about the common cold is that contact with bacteria is the main cause when in fact the cause is contact with a virus, which makes the run to get antibiotics almost pointless. There is no cure for the common cold, but one trick when you begin to feel sick is a few drops of 3% hydrogen peroxide into each ear. Once the bubbling and slight stinging subside (around 5-10 minutes), drain onto a tissue.*

If you have a cold or flu, try 3% hydrogen peroxide. It's easy, it's inexpensive, and you can find it at almost any drug store near you.

Toxic Dental Fillings

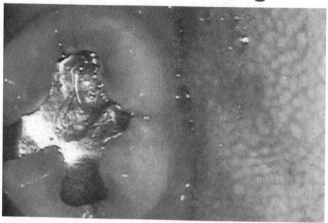

A single dental amalgam filling releases as much as 15 micrograms of mercury per day, which is absorbed directly into your body.* This can cause permanent damage to the brain, kidneys, immune, neurological and gastrointestinal systems. The Canadian government advised dentists to stop placing amalgam in children and pregnant women in 1996 -- nearly 15 years ago! Denmark, Norway and Sweden have essentially banned amalgams. But in the United States, they're still regarded as the "gold standard" of dental care.

If you have dental amalgam fillings in your mouth, check your blood for high heavy metal counts. You may have to have these amalgam fillings removed and replace them with ceramic fillings.

Pain Medicine Darvon/Darvocet Pulled off the Market

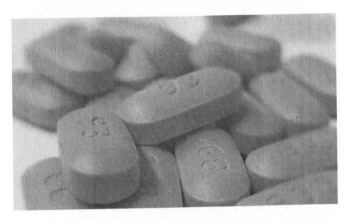

Documentation shows that deaths from prescribed prescription medications is the cause of death for over 100,000 Americans annually.* The makers of Darvon/Darvocet pulled these two products off the shelves, including generic brands, by order of the FDA. The safety risks it posed to patients were symptoms from irregular heart rhythms to Britain's ban on the drug because of suicides and accidental overdoses.** Proposyphene is the main ingredient in these drugs that has been known to cause accidental overdoses.

Stay away from these types of pain medications! Try a holistic herbal pain relief such as ginger, turmeric, rhodiola, chamomile and peppermint.

Powerful Pomegranate Juice

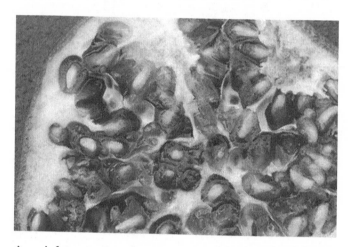

An eight-ounce glass of pomegranate juice provides about 50% of an adult's recommended daily allowance (RDA) of the vitamins A, C and E, 100% RDA of folic acid, and 13% RDA of potassium.* Research has shown this fruit juice may help reduce the risk of prostate and breast cancer and heart disease. It also can lower serum cholesterol and protect arteries from clogging. This wonder juice may also inhibit viral infections and have antibacterial effects against dental plaque.

Juice a pomegranate fruit today. Enjoy the health effect of this powerful fruit.

The Foot, an Amazing Walking Machine

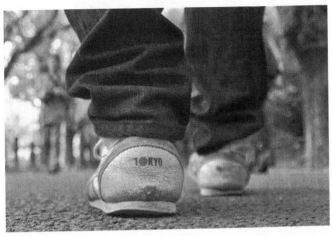

Your foot has 26 bones, 33 joints, 107 ligaments, 20 muscles, 7,000 nerve endings and 250,000 sweat glands. The average person will walk more than 250,000 miles in a lifetime. While walking, your foot will absorb twice the amount of your body weight whereas running will make your foot absorb two and a half times your weight.*

Let's appreciate our feet. They do so much work every day carrying us where we need to go. Let's take care of them by wearing proper shoes and arch supports when necessary.

Do Not Compromise Sleep

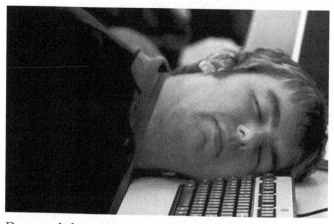

Research has shown that the quantity and quality of sleep we get each night has the potential to affect our health, our productivity on the job and our ability to concentrate and function while attempting even the most routine activities.* The average adult requires seven to nine hours of sleep each night. Babies and younger children need a greater amount of sleep than adults. The elderly, although requiring less sleep, are often victims of poor quality rest.

You don't start your day in the morning. You actually launch your day at night by preparing with sleep. Do not compromise your sleep. The lack of rest will compromise every aspect of your life.

Male Menopause

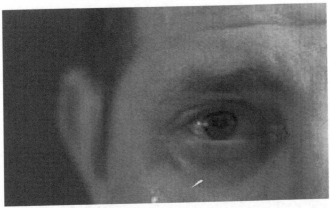

While some physicians scoff at the concept of male menopause, there is no question that testosterone production slows down around age 40 and steadily declines thereafter. This decline may be marked by decreasing sexual performance or interest in sex. A trial of bioidentical testosterone replacement can help. In addition to pronounced effects on sex, testosterone replacement therapy improves bone density, muscle mass, body composition, mood, energy, cognitive function, cardiovascular health, and quality of life. Furthermore, it reduces the risk of diabetes and heart disease.

Bioidentical testosterone is provided through 200 mg injections of testosterone cypionate every seven to 10 days or daily applications of testosterone creams or gels. These are all available from compounding pharmacies.*

Goji Berries for Your Health

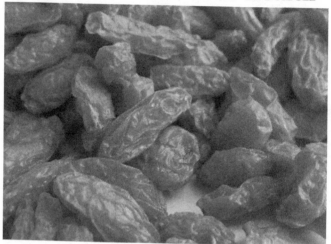

Wolfberries, commercially called Goji berries, contain an abundance of naturally occurring minerals such as Zinc, Germanium, Selenium, Iron, Copper and Phosphorus. Goji Berries contain 19 amino acids and the Linoleic acid (Essential Omega 6 fat) that promotes the loss of body fat. They also have plenty of antioxidants and phytonutrients that reduce age-related macular degeneration, boost immune system and reduce fatigue. In addition, they improve eyesight, great hair color, improved libido, improvement in mood, more quality sleep, and enhanced energy levels.*

Try Goji berries as tea, as juice or in soups. You can also chew on dried Goji berries and enjoy the great taste.

Get a Massage

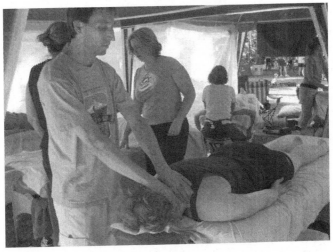

Massage offers many health benefits. Massage increases circulation, reduces tightness in muscles, stimulates the release of pain-relieving endorphins and lowers stress hormone levels. It is also known to enhance serotonin, a well-known contributor to feelings of well-being.* It prevents fibrosis or scar tissue, improves sleep, and reduces anxiety and depression.

Get a massage today. Try different forms of massage that you never experienced before. How did you feel afterward?

Perform a Shoe Test

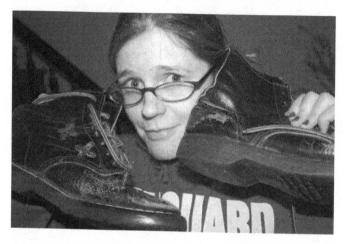

Bad shoes account for about 90% of all foot problems. No matter what type of shoe you are wearing make sure that the heel counter is stiff and firm upon squeezing, the arch is firm and should not twist easily, the ball of the shoes should bend to allow your feet to naturally roll over, and the more cushion and traction on the outer sole of the shoes the better.*

Next time you purchase a pair of shoes, perform a shoe test. Squeeze the heel counter, twist the arch and bend at the ball of the shoes.

No More Fluoride Products

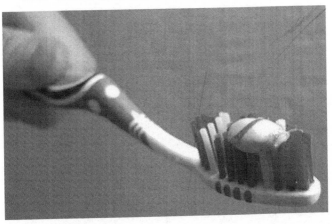

A new study from the Journal of the American Dental Association finds that contrary to what most people have been told, fluoride is actually bad for teeth.* Exposure to high levels of fluoride results in a condition known as fluorosis, in which tooth enamel becomes discolored. The condition can eventually lead to badly damaged teeth. The new study found that fluoride intake during a child's first few years of life is significantly associated with fluorosis, and warned against using fluoridated water in infant formula.

Do not drink tap water, which has fluoride. Do not use fluoride products such as fluoride tooth paste, fluoride mouth rinse, fluoride supplements, fluoride gel and foam and fluoride varnish. Make sure you read the labels.

Schedule Downtime First

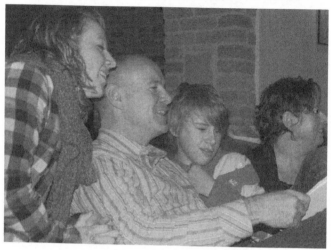

When you're overloaded by activity, you're in survival mode, just trying to make it through another day. If you feel you are too busy to respond to your loved ones when they ask you for a favor, you've lost a great opportunity to connect with them.

Schedule downtime before you schedule your activities. You will enjoy your day more and your loved ones will appreciate it.

Hyperbaric Oxygen Therapy

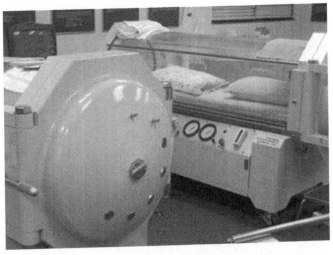

The safety and efficacy of hyperbaric oxygen treatment for almost 200 diverse conditions has been demonstrated in tens of thousands of scientific studies published over the past 70 years. Hyperbaric oxygen treats slow-healing ulcers and other wounds, improves circulation, aids in stroke rehabilitation, helps with heart disease, cures carbon monoxide poisoning, chronic fatigue and multiple pain syndromes and cuts post-surgery healing time in half.*

If you have the conditions listed above, look into getting a hyperbaric oxygen therapy. Your body is crying out for more oxygen.

Avoid Eating in Front of the TV or Computer

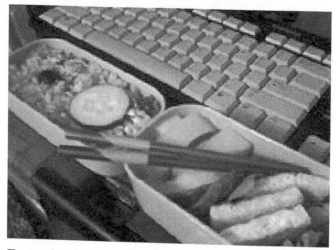

By eating your meal in front of the TV or computer your brain becomes distracted and it can lose track of how much you have taken in, which will result in overindulgence. In addition, people who were distracted during their meal felt hungry again thirty minutes later, thus eating twice as much than people who ate without distraction.*

Take your meal to the table. Eat in peace and without distraction from your TV or computer and see the benefits in your waistline.

Walk for Your Brain

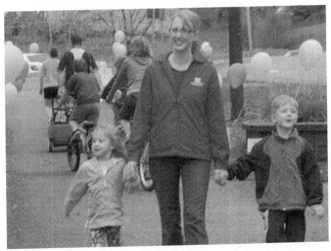

Brain size shrinks in late adulthood, which can cause dementia and Alzheimer's disease. According to a study published by the medical journal of the American Academy of Neurology, walking at least six miles per week may protect brain size and in turn, preserve memory in old age. Researchers found that those who walked the most cut their risk of developing memory problems in half.*

Walking is the best aerobic exercise which oxygenates your brain. Take deep breaths while walking and feel the oxygen getting to your brain cells.

Peppermint Oil for Better Digestion

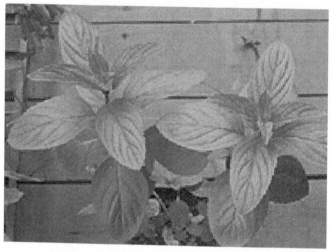

Peppermint oil has many health benefits that include treating indigestion, respiratory problems, headache, nausea, fever, stomach, IBS (Irritable Bowel Syndrome), gas, motion sickness, heartburn (when used in combination with caraway oil) and pain.

Peppermint oil also contains minerals and nutrients that include manganese, iron, magnesium, calcium, folate, potassium, copper as well as omega-3 fatty acids, and vitamins A and C.* Take two capsules of peppermint oil per day especially if you have digestion problems.

Dehydrated Kids

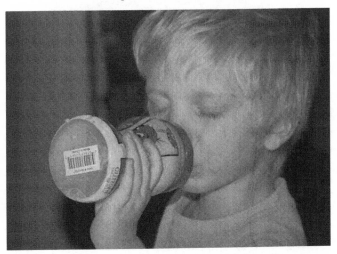

When your kids feel light-headed, tired and nauseous, they are already too dehydrated. Kids are more vulnerable to dehydration than adults.* They don't sweat as much as adults so they cannot cool their body as efficiently. Encourage them to get in the habit of having more water throughout the day.

Remind your kids to drink more water through-out the day and have more fruits in-between meals to hydrate them instead of salty or oily snacks. Discourage them from drinking artificial energy drinks or soda, which will just dehydrate them more.

Frequent Smaller Meals

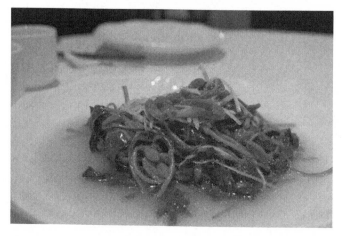

Eating smaller meals throughout the day will help kick start your metabolism, hence the weight loss. The constant rate of energy consumed will help in keeping the fire of your metabolism burning throughout the day. Eating frequent smaller meals takes your body off the sugar roller coaster ride, which becomes a big stress relief for your body.*

Remember that when your body is stressed, it tends to retain fat. Focus on eating five or six small meals a day which will help your energy to soar and weight to reduce.

Energy Drinks Make You Fat

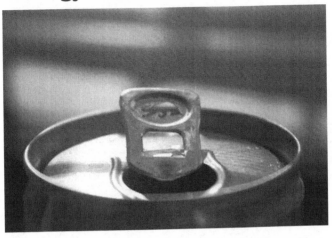

Containing large amounts of caffeine and artificially- derived vitamins and sugar (high fructose corn syrup), energy drinks are packed with calories that will add to your waistline as well as cause nervousness, irritability, increased heart rate and insomnia. Energy drinks only supply extra calories and convenience, not the ability to run faster or manage weight.*

Let's stop drinking energy drinks. They may give you a short burst of energy, but they are very fattening. Water is always your best choice for keeping you strong and hydrated.

Avoid These Skin Products

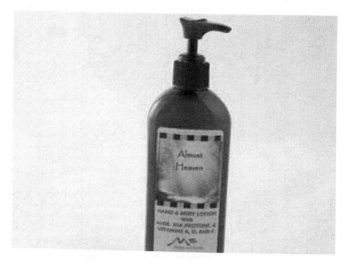

Your skin is only 1/10th of an inch thick and highly permeable to every toxin around. The following ingredients in the skin products can cause dermatitis, cancer, kidney and liver disease, and anemia: Parabens, Mineral Oil, Paraffin, and Petrolatum, Sodium Laureth Sulfate, Acrylamide, Propylene glycol, Phenol carbolic acid, Dioxane and Toluene.*

Go grab your containers of skin care products and check out what you're putting on your skin. If these ingredients are listed, stay away from them!

Sitting Causes Flat Feet

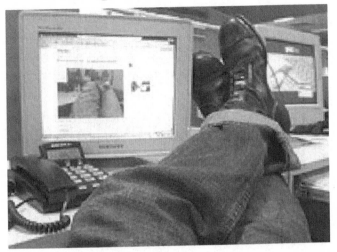

Fallen arches affect roughly 70% of the population, due to a sedentary lifestyle. On average, Americans sit for 10 hours per day. Sitting causes your hamstring (back of your thighs) muscles to tighten up, which causes your hip to tilt forward putting extra pressure on the balls of your feet. This will cause your feet to over-pronate, or roll more inward than normal, causing your arches to fall.*

Avoid sitting for too long. Take frequent walking breaks to offset these ill effects and stretch your hamstrings by bending forward to touch your toes.

Benefits of Black Cherries

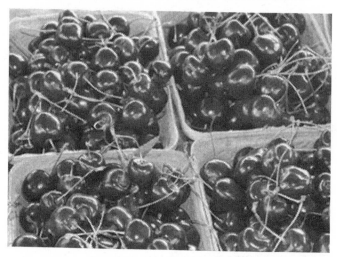

Black cherries have some of the highest anti-oxidant potency of all fruits and vegetables. They inhibit an enzyme called xanthine oxidase, a major source of harmful free radicals. Research has shown them to be highly beneficial as an anti-inflammatory in gout and arthritis treatment, in the prevention of muscle damage, protection from cancer and heart diseases as well as a great sleep aide.*

Let's snack on black cherries, which are a great source of vitamins and powerful antioxidants that fight many diseases.

Vary Your Exercises

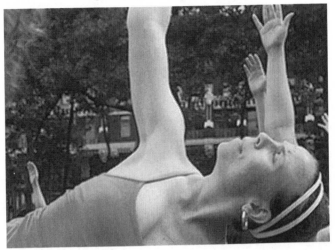

Too often, people get bored with their exercise programs and abandon them. If you feel bored, ask yourself if you've been doing the same exercises at the same speed, order and repetition.*

Vary your exercises to avoid this pitfall. Consider weight training, jog, cycle, swim, walk, yoga, Pilates classes, dance and tennis. Vary the speed, order and length of your exercises.

Custom Foot Orthotics

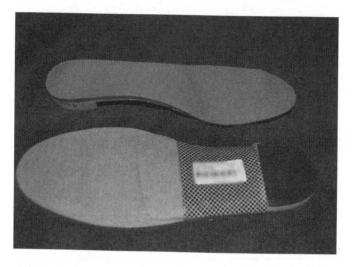

Between 70-85% of people have biomechanical imperfections, but not all need orthotic control. About 90% of people over-pronate (results in fallen arches) and about 4% are over-supinators (results in high arches). The imbalance of your feet can cause ankle, knee, hip, back, and neck pain. Custom foot orthotics are custom made arch supports that balance your feet to give you better posture, which will improve your ability to walk and stand with less pain.*

If you have pain on your feet, ankle, knee, back, and neck, have your feet checked by a foot specialist. You may benefit from custom foot orthotics.

Empty Calories for Children

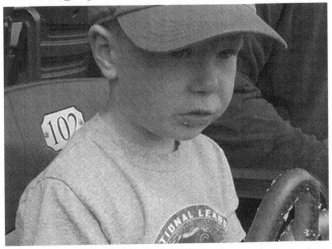

According to the Journal of the American Dietetic Association, 40 percent of calories in children's diets are so-called "empty calories," that do not provide any nutritional value. A large percentage of these empty calories come from sugar-sweetened drinks, such as fruit juice and soda as well as cookies, pizza, and yeast breads.*

Because of excessive weight gain associated with high consumption of sugary drinks, they should be avoided by your children at all cost. Keep your children away from those drinks and foods of empty calories. Replace them with spring water and vegetables.

Tell Others "Non-GMO"

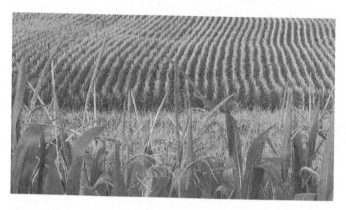

A genetically modified organism (GMO) has been altered scientifically using genetic engineering techniques such as Monsanto's "Roundup Ready" soybeans. Studies have linked GMO foods to increased risk of cancer, food allergies, accelerated aging, immune system damage and susceptibility to super viruses. Eight major GMO food crops on the market: soy, corn, cottonseed (used in vegetable cooking oils), canola (canola oil), sugar beets, Hawaiian papaya, and some varieties of zucchini crookneck squash. The European Union has banned use GMO products, due to the unknown risks of long-term consumption.*

Tell others about the risks of GMO foods. When you buy food, look for "non-GMO" labels. Support the non-GMO movement by going to nongmoproject.org and responsibletechnology.org

Body Fat and Breast Cancer

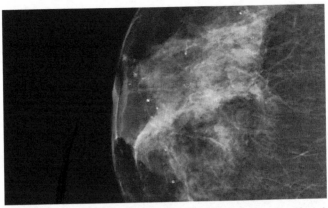

The risk of breast cancer is related to obesity.* Fat cells produce estrogen in addition to the ovaries. After menopause, fat becomes the primary site where estrogen is manufactured in your body. Higher levels of insulin and insulin-like growth factor-1 (IGF-1), also linked to obesity, significantly increase breast cancer risk. About 20 to 30 percent of all postmenopausal breast cancers are thought to be caused primarily by obesity.

Reduce your fat percentage by doing resistance exercises such as weight training. When you increase your muscles, they burn more fat naturally.

Exercise and Colds

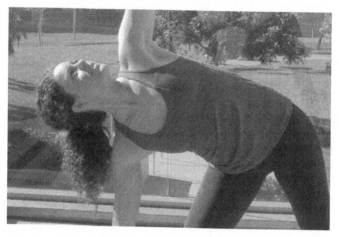

The average American adult suffers from two to four colds a year, which add up to approximately 1 billion colds per year in the United States. The latest study showed that exercise cuts the risk of having a cold by 50 percent, and cuts the severity of symptoms by 31 percent among those who did catch a cold. The researchers noted that each round of exercise may lead to a boost in circulating immune system cells that could help ward off a cold virus.*

Exercise regularly to ward off colds. Increase frequency and length of exercise during the flu season.

Indoor Heating
will Dry You Out!

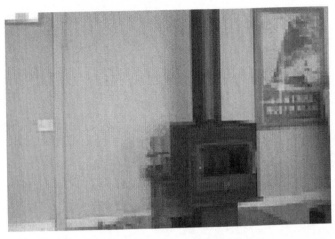

Dry skin is especially common in winter because the humidity levels outside drop and your skin is unable to hold as much moisture. The warm, dry indoor heating may feel nice, but it actually dries out your skin more, as well as your mucous membranes, your lips become chapped, dry noses will lead to nosebleeds, and your dry throat will give you that infamous winter sore throat.*

When the heat is on, set it to the lowest comfortable temperature; use a humidifier or place an oven-safe pan of water over a radiator as needed to keep the air moist and healthy for your skin.

Respond to Your Calling

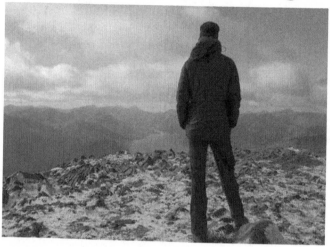

You were sent to this world to carry out your ultimate calling by God.* Everyone is called by God according to his or her ambition, value, talent, experience or passion. Some of this calling may be difficult and other parts may be easy. In either case, the work is significant. Each element of the work helps creates something great for the future.

What is your calling in life? Think about your ambition, value, talent, experience or passion. Contribute to a greater future by responding to your calling today.

Take Deep Breaths

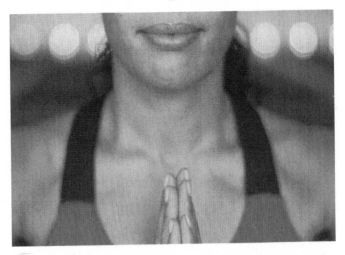

Taking deep breaths not only calms the mind, but has other health benefits such as: lowering blood pressure, slowing the heart rate, relaxing muscles, reduces insomnia and anxiety, increases energy, and is also very beneficial to the lymphatic system. Every part of our body relies on oxygen and when you take a deep breath, you are allowing more oxygen to enter the body and more toxins to leave.*

Take a moment during your busy day and inhale deep through your nose and out through your mouth. Take three deep breaths at a time. You will feel the benefits!

How to be a Centenarian

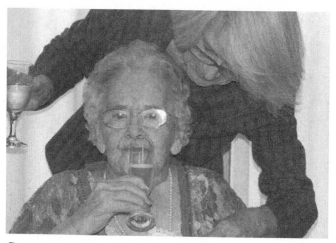

Centenarians are still a bit rare, but according to recent research they are growing in numbers. There were an estimated 50,454 centenarians in 2000 and by 2050 there is an expected growth to number more than 800,000. So, what's the secret? Genes and healthy living are definitely factors, but the surprising factors are attitude and personality. How centenarians reacted to life stresses and changes as well as keeping a happy open mind made the difference to gaining some years.*

Let's keep an attitude of happiness and take things lightly to live healthfully for a hundred years. Laugh often and don't let life get a negative hold on you.

How to Drop
52 Pounds a Year

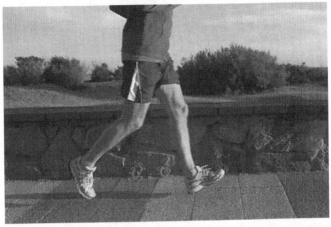

When you walk 10,000 steps (5 miles) a day, you will burn 500 calories. If you walk 7 days a week, you will burn 3,500 calories per week. This is equivalent to one pound of fat loss per week. If you do this for 52 weeks, you will drop 52 pounds per year!*

Increase your steps slowly to reach 10,000 steps a day while soaking up the sun and getting some fresh air. Use a pedometer to count your steps and watch as your health dramatically improves.

Power of Love

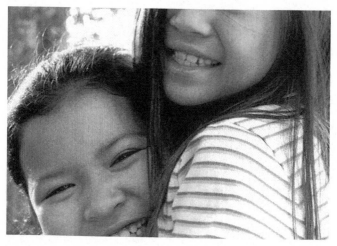

"Power is of two kinds. One is obtained by the fear of punishment and the other by acts of love. Power based on love is a thousand times more effective and permanent than the one derived from fear of punishment." -Mahatma Gandhi

Think of all the things you love to do, and do more of them. You will feel the power of love when you do.

Foot Care During Pregnancy

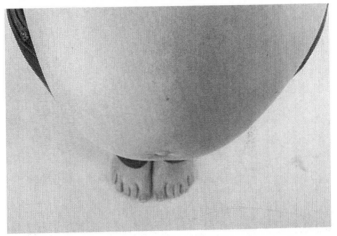

Weight gain and postural changes during pregnancy can lead to uncomfortable problems such as foot and leg fatigue, over-pronation and edema. Over-pronation or flat foot is caused when the feet roll inward by the weight gain. Edema, or swelling, occurs because of the extra volume of blood circulating through the body. Be on the look out if the swelling isn't symmetrical. This could be a sign of a vascular problem and a doctor should be informed immediately.*

Proper shoes that are flexible to allow for changes in foot size and proper arch support should be a priority. In addition, keep hydrated, keep your feet elevated, wear seamless socks to allow for circulation, and stretch often.

Benefits of Qigong

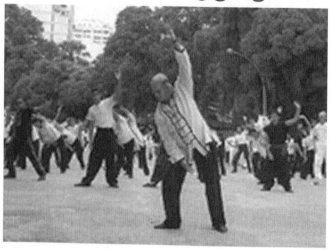

Called the mother of Chinese healing, Qigong is one of the cornerstones of traditional Chinese medicine. Qi, meaning vital breath or life energy, and Gong, meaning to cultivate or practice, come together to form medicine that uses breath control and slow, relaxed motions to increase the circulation of Qi in the body. This form of deep breathing has many health benefits such as providing oxygen to cells, blood and organs; relieving tension in muscles, slows the heart rate and quiets the mind.*

Incorporate Qigong into your lifestyle and restore balance between your mental and physical well-being. By acquiring this skill, you will help your body's Qi to promote health and healing.

Use Headsets

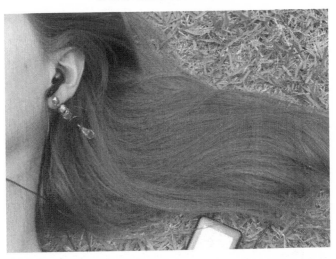

The need for cell phone connection will eventually cause problems for your back and neck. Holding a phone for an extended period of time causes constant tension in your neck muscles that will adapt to their shortened position in cradling the phone. When your call ends and your arm lowers, these muscles will continue to be partially contracted until they're stretched out. In addition to this, you have cranial nerves that could get compressed, which gives you that "pinched nerve" feeling.*

Prevent back and neck pain by getting a headset for your phone! They provide benefits in posture as well as giving you the freedom to do other tasks with both hands.

Energetic Beets

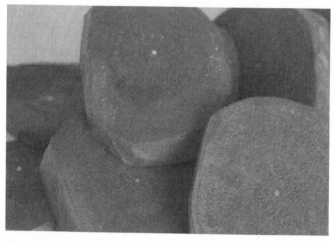

Beets are members of the Chenopodiaceae (Goosefoot) Family. Beets, being round roots are said to have a downward energy, affecting the lower organs and especially benefiting the colon, kidneys, bladder, spleen and liver. They are considered a fiber food containing sodium, magnesium, calcium, iron, phosphorous, and vitamins A and C; they are a great source for folic acid and they protect against cancer and heart disease.*

Try beets grated raw into a salad. Season with a bit of honey and lemon. A beautiful beet soup, known as borscht is hearty and delicious. Seasonings that bring out the best in beets include dill weed, basil, parsley and tarragon.

Dr. S. Don Kim

Go Organic Carefully

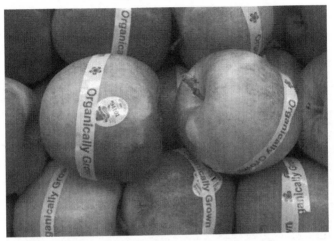

Going organic is great, but be careful because not all labels mean "organic." According to the USDA, the "organic" label must meet the following criteria: produced without harmful pesticides, fertilizers that contain synthetic ingredients, and without ionizing radiation. For meat: no growth hormones or antibiotics used on the animal. Now in contrast, the label "natural" has only the regulation in reference to meat: does not contain artificial ingredients or added color and has minimal processing.*

Watch out when you buy "organic." Slapping labels on products to claim that they are "all-natural" can be used as a marketing tool because of the "organic" demand. Read your labels and purchase organic foods carefully.

189

Orthotics for Calluses

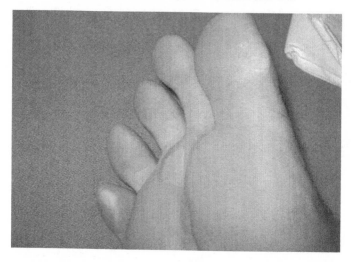

Calluses are formed as a defense against excessive pressure and friction on an area of the foot. Dead skin cells accumulate and thicken over time forming a hard cover over the area. Though this is a method of the body protecting itself, it can do harm by causing pain or pressure. Common causes of calluses are: high-heeled shoes, tight shoes, obesity, irregular walking motions, flat feet, and high arches.*

See your foot doctor for special orthotics that will equally redistribute weight and move pressure away from the effected areas. Home remedies for calluses are as easy as soaking your feet and using a pumice stone to reduce the size of the callus.

Don't Shop Hungry

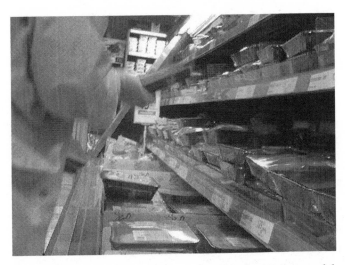

Do not go to the grocery store hungry! It's an old saying, but there's more value in it today than ever before. People want healthy lifestyles and a growing budget, but shopping when you're hungry will sabotage both. If you're starving, which looks better to buy and satisfy your craving: a glazed doughnut or a whole-wheat muffin? Furthermore, since you are trying to satisfy your cravings and buy healthy your pocket book will suffer because you will end up purchasing more by the end of the trip.*

Eat a healthy snack before you shop! When you're satisfied you will stick to your list making healthy choices and keeping money in your wallet.

Avoid Guilt and Resentment

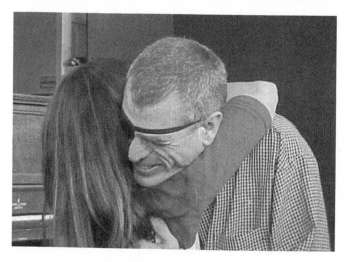

You will never reach the goals you set in your life if you're carrying the extra baggage of guilt and resentment. They slow you down. Ask for forgiveness when you hurt others and offer forgiveness to those who have hurt you. This will free you to move forward. However, if you let go of the resentment and forgive others, but don't forgive yourself then you'll still be carrying the baggage of guilt that will keep you from reaching your goals!

Let both guilt and resentment go by practicing forgiveness! Forgive others and yourself. Remember forgiveness is freedom!

Ask for Help

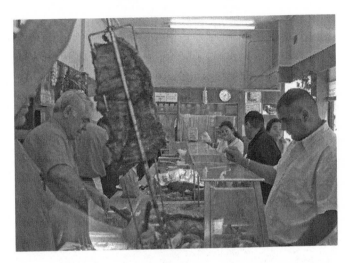

Around 1997 there were around 7,200 meat markets and just four years later it shrunk to 6,042. Americans love to get things quickly and that even means shopping quickly. Don't forget your butcher! Talking to your butcher can really help in achieving a healthy lifestyle. Butchers are very knowledgeable about the meats they serve. Whatever you are looking for they can recommend the best product, cut, portion size and even the best way to cook it for your desired meal.*

Go to the meat counter! Don't be intimidated to talk to your local butcher. The assistance you get will yield the best and most healthy possibilities for your meal.

Must Take Supplements for Diabetics

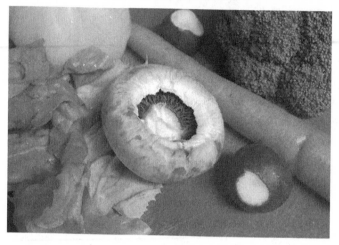

Nearly 24 million Americans suffer from diabetes. Worldwide this condition is expected to double from 171 million in 2000 to 366 million in 2030. This is truly an epidemic. Fortunately, 90% of this disease can be treated and prevented with weight loss, proper diet, exercise and supplementation.*

You must lose weight by proper diet and exercise if you want to improve your diabetes. To fight against complications of the blood vessels, nerves, eyes and kidneys, you must supplement with vanadyl sulfate, alpha lipoic acid, chromium, cinnamon and Gymnema sylvestre.

Watch Out for a Stress Fracture in your Foot

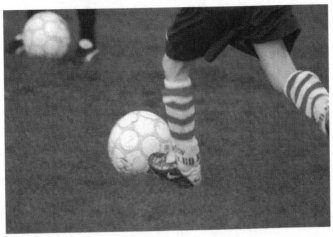

High stresses, strong forces and high impact sporting activity landings can lead to a stress fracture. The most common symptoms are swelling and sensitivity on the ball of the foot around the second toe. You may think men have more problems with getting a stress fracture, but it's actually women who hold the higher percentage. Factors like eating disorders, amenorrhea (irregular periods), and osteoporosis add to the likelihood of women receiving a stress fracture.*

Lessen your chances of getting a stress fracture foot by having the proper shoe support, slowly increasing your activity levels, and changing up your exercise routine.

Avoid Perfectionism

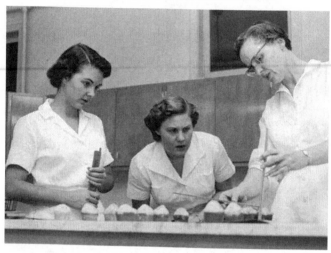

When you frequently say "I should", "I must", or "I have to", you are most likely a perfectionist. Perfectionists are hard on themselves and can be difficult to work with. This is because nothing is good enough for them and they project their dissatisfaction and blame it on themselves.

Focus on a few things in your life that you want to remain perfect. Regularly remind yourself that it is fine to do other things in a less-than-perfect manner. Being a perfectionist is very dangerous for your health and well being by causing stress and worry. Find the perfection in who you already are.

Meat as Side Dishes

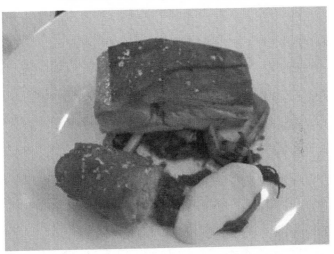

A meat-based diet, or meat as a main dish diet, is high in saturated fat, which your body converts to cholesterol. Such diets are also high in iron, an oxidant that makes cholesterol more likely to clog your arteries. Iron also causes the formation of free radicals, which promotes cancer and aging.* A meat-based diet is low in antioxidants that help prevent this from occurring.

Rather than having meat as a main dish, try meat as a side dish of plant based foods. Try chicken salad or fish salad. Use vegetables as the main course and sprinkle meat over the vegetables.

Lead Your Children by Example

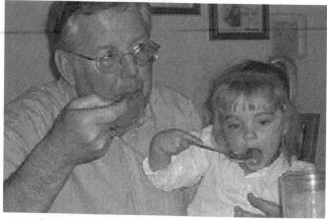

It is during a child's formative years that health habits become ingrained. Food preferences, exercise and play routines, TV-watching patterns, and emotional responses are all learned behaviors that will follow your children into adulthood. Children might not be very good at listening to their parents, but they have never failed to imitate them. Your examples are far more compelling than your words.

Make your health habits positive ones. Your children will follow. Remember, they are fast learners.

Tragic Trans Fats

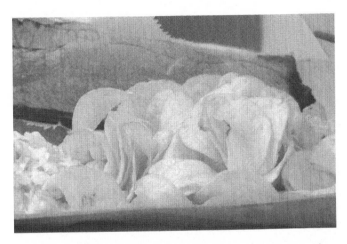

Trans fats (hydrogenated fats) became popular in the middle of the 20th century as a way to prolong the shelf life of packaged foods. When this chemical process transforms liquid vegetable oil into a solid substance, they preserve them for months without refrigeration. Almost all packaged goods have been processed this way. Trans fats are linked to arterial plaque formation, cancer, diabetes, obesity, Alzheimer's disease, liver dysfunction and infertility in women.*

Read the label of packaged foods and look for "hydrogenated oil" or "partially hydrogenated oil". Avoid these trans fats at all costs for optimal health.

Buddy Splint Your Toes

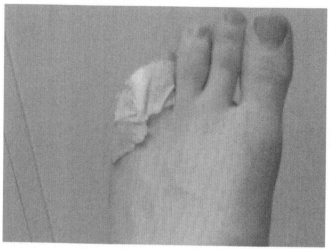

You're walking through the house with no lights on...and it happens! You stub your toe. Whether the toe is broken or not, the proper way to aid your toe is to apply a buddy splint. This involves wrapping gauze around the broken, or injured, toe and the next biggest toe that is not injured. Place a popsicle stick or cotton ball between the toes so the injured one heals straight. Apply medical tape to hold the gauze in place.*

Do not ignore symptoms! If the swelling and pain does not subside in three days, you need to visit your foot doctor in case the injured toe is broken.

Krill Oil Lowers Cholesterol

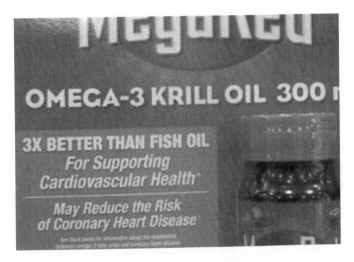

Krill, the tiny, shrimp-like crustaceans plentiful in every ocean, are a primary food for many marine animals. Recent research showed that one to three grams of krill oil outperformed fish oil and placebo for lowering bad cholesterol and increasing good cholesterol. It also fights chronic inflammation linked to heart disease, stroke, Alzheimer's disease and Rheumatoid arthritis.*

Krill oil can be purchased from several online retailers or found in health food stores. If you have one of the above conditions, give Krill oil a try.

Are You Watching Too Much TV?

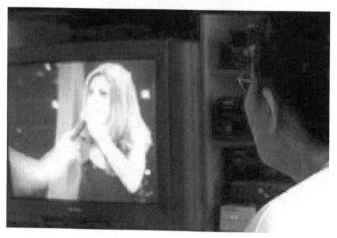

The average American watches nearly five hours of TV every day. Watching TV is linked to obesity, decreased metabolism, eyesight damage, decreased attention span, hormonal disturbances, autism, sleep difficulties, limited brain growth and diabetes.* The worst part, though, is all of the negative images and gratuitous violence that is so common on TV.

Limit your TV time. Only watch positive and uplifting shows. Try fasting-no TV at all-for one whole week and see how you feel.

Smart Snacks

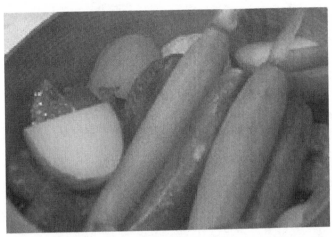

Snacking, or eating small meals throughout the day, is crucial to keep your blood sugar level constant. If you find yourself feeling very hungry, your blood sugar levels have already dropped too low, which can cause you to overeat. Instead of sugary, starchy, and fat-laden treats, choose snacks that provide protein and fiber. Unlike carbohydrates, which the body burns quickly for fuel, protein and fiber provide slow-burning energy and help you feel full longer.*

Almonds, sunflower seeds, edamame, celery ribs with almond butter, low fat cottage cheese, hard boiled eggs, protein shakes and steamed vegetables all make great smart snacks. Don't go hungry. Get smart.

Don't Say "Try"

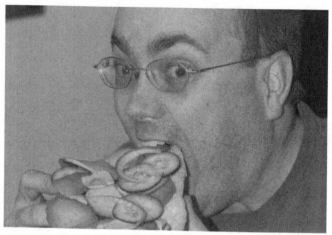

I will try to drink more water. I will try to eat more vegetables. I will try to quit coffee. I will try to eat less junk food. I will try to exercise three times a week. I will try to think only positive thoughts from now on. I will try to stop mindless internet surfing. I will try to laugh more.

When you say "try", you give the impression that you have an excuse to fail. You will see better results if you simply express what you will do.

Cure for Athlete's Foot

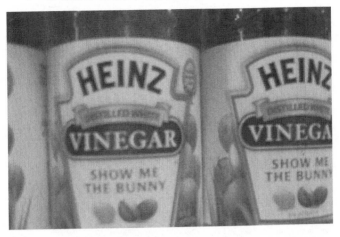

Around 70% of people will have Athlete's foot at some point in their lives. Athlete's foot is a fungus, called trichophyton, most commonly found between your toes. It thrives in warm, moist areas such as locker rooms, showers and swimming pools. Symptoms of Athlete's foot are: dry skin, pain, itching, scaling, inflammation, burning and stinging sensations as well as blisters. Watch out for blisters! If left untreated they can be a breeding ground for more infections.*

Soak your feet in 2 tablespoons of organic vinegar or organic salt mixed with warm water for 15 minutes every night. Apply baking soda paste to the affected area for 1-2 hours, then rinse, dry and dust with cornstarch. Continue until fungus passes.

Plant-based Diet

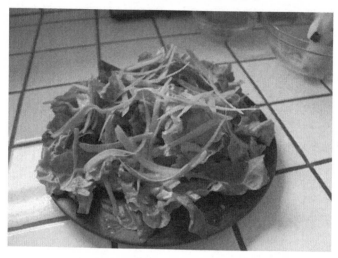

A plant based diet is linked not only to lower rates of heart disease and stroke, but also to significantly lower rates of the most common cancers. These include colon and lung cancers, prostate cancer in men and breast and ovarian cancers in women. This diet may also reduce the incidence of osteoporosis, adult-onset diabetes, hypertension, obesity and many other chronic illnesses.*

At least half of your plate should be vegetables. They are rich in Vitamin A, C, E, and antioxidants. It will help your health and the fiber in the vegetables will help enhance your digestive power.

Plan Your Meals with a List

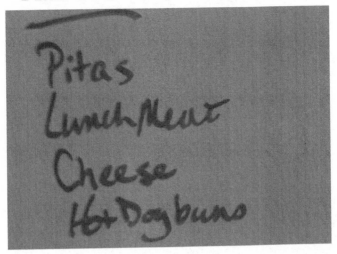

Want to streamline your shopping experience, save money and eat healthier? Spend one day to plan your meals for that week. Here are four easy steps to help: keep a running tab on what's in your fridge, gather your recipes, plan your meals and make your master grocery list. By knowing what you have in the fridge you will see quicker what items you need from the recipes you pick out. Make your list and watch your grocery shopping take less time.*

Spend a day to plan your meals! Planning your meals will help alleviate food waste, keep down your food costs, and make dinner that much easier each night.

Little Faith, Big Worries

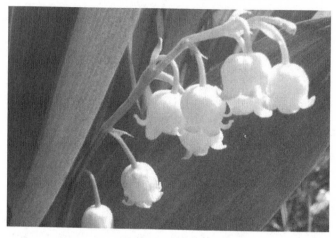

"Look at the lilies and how they grow...if God cares so wonderfully for flowers that are here today and gone tomorrow, won't he more surely care for you? You have so little faith! "
- Matthew 6:28-30.

Worry works on us; it doesn't work for us. It creates more difficulties than you need. Choose faith instead! Then your worries will diminish.

Try Health Food Stores

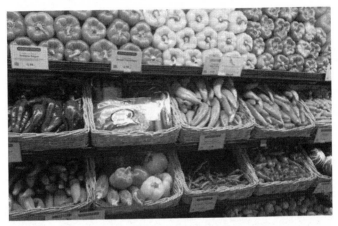

It's a battle between quick and easy and staying healthy. Since people don't have time to run to different stores to try and get the healthiest foods, try a health food store such as Henry's or Whole Foods. Stores like these will give you all your grocery needs while providing a great selection of healthy choices. There is also the option of trying an online Health Food store such as wholefoodsmarket.com or shoporganic.com. It just takes a few moments to start your shopping online and click for pick-up or delivery.*

Try a health food store! Shopping at health food stores can turn into your one-stop-shop for all your health needs. The online option is great to get all your needs organized in less time.

Trim Your Toenails Correctly

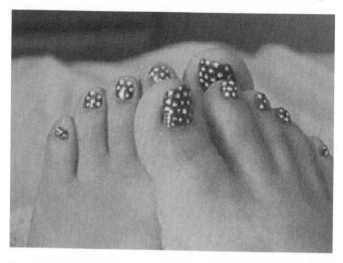

Onychocryptosis, or ingrown toenail, is a very common problem. You can fix this by trimming your toenail correctly. First, use toenail clippers and not fingernail clippers because they are meant to handle the thicker nail. Second, always cut straight across and never down the sides. Third, do not tear the nail. This will cause sensitivity and infection. Fourth, always cut dry and in small cuts. And lastly, do not cut all the way down for this can also cause infection from sensitivity and shoe pressure.*

Avoid a surgical procedure and cut those nails properly. You depend on your feet everyday, so take care of them!

Dr. S. Don Kim

Get your Beauty Sleep

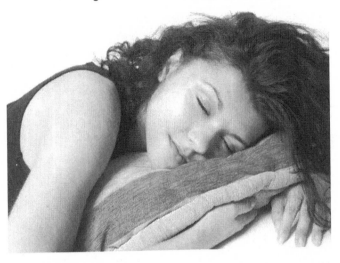

"A good rest has always been called beauty sleep. No beauty cream, no facials, no amount of makeup can give you the glow, fresh and relaxed look that a sound whole beauty sleep provides." The average adult needs to have at least 7 hours of sleep per 24 hours. Think about this: the skin makes new cells twice as fast during sleep time than when you are awake. When you don't get enough sleep, your face will appear dry, fatigued, and your muscle tone will appear slack.*

Get your beauty sleep! It's the easiest beauty tip out there. Focus on a good nights sleep and you will appear fresh and younger every morning.

More Fiber in the Morning

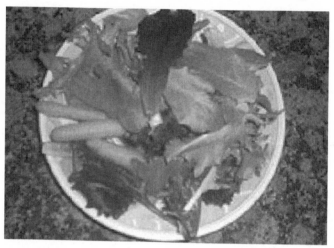

"A great way to kick-start your metabolism in the morning is to add fiber to your breakfast! Fiber slows your digestive system down which means you will feel full longer and it slows the rate at which sugars enter your body. This will prevent spikes in blood sugar and keep your levels, as well as mood swings, even throughout the day. In addition to bumping your metabolism up, when fiber is broken down in your colon it will create acids that will provide fuel for your liver.*

Add some fiber to your morning meal. This can be a great way to start off the day with better eating habits that lead to a healthier lifestyle.

Amazing Chestnuts

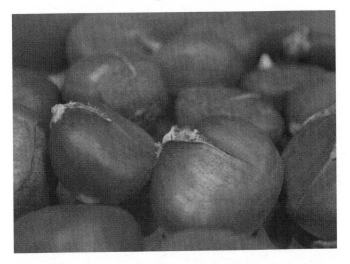

Besides being a holiday staple, the chestnut is an amazing little nut that packs a nutritional punch. Chestnuts are low in fat (containing less than 1 gm in one chestnut) with a good amount of fiber, manganese, potassium, copper, phosphorus, magnesium, iron, zinc, and calcium. They also contain a culmination of vitamin C, vitamin B6, and vitamin A. Like other nuts, they help in preventing heart risks, they provide energy, and are low in cholesterol.*

Chestnuts are great additions to cooking, whether sweet or savory. Try crumbling a few of these on your next dish and reap the benefits and flavor!

Benefits of
Shiitake Mushrooms

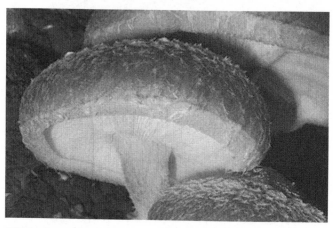

Shiitake mushrooms have long been revered in Japan for their cancer fighting properties. They contain a complex sugar called lentinan. When you eat shiitake mushrooms your immune system goes in overdrive creating infection-fighting cells. Research has discovered that when people with tumors are fed a dried mushroom powder containing lentinan, they can inhibit tumor growth by 70 percent. These powerful properties are now being studied for the fight against HIV.*

Add these dark meaty mushrooms to your meals! They make a great addition to soups, stews and vegetable dishes.

Rheumatoid Arthritis and Your Feet

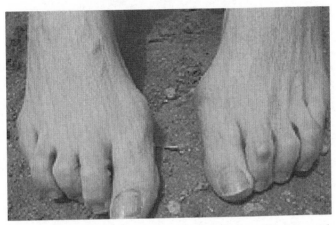

About 90% of people who have been diagnosed with rheumatoid arthritis will develop symptoms in their feet. Rheumatoid arthritis is a disease that attacks your own immune system. Instead of protecting your joints, your body will attack and inflame your joints causing pain, swelling, and stiffness. When it comes to your feet, you could develop bunions and your toes may begin to curl causing issues such as claw or hammer toe.*

If you have been diagnosed with Rheumatoid arthritis, you should see a podiatrist right away. You need custom molded shoes and insoles to prevent further subluxation of the joints of your feet and ankle.

Avoid Eyestrain

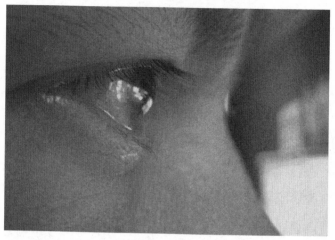

Over the last 50 years our focus of vision has been reduced to arm's length because of computer work, recreation and video games. These changes can produce eyestrain, nearsightedness and suppressed vision. Computer users experience visual stress because of an increase in the number and complexity of eye movements and focus skills, poor lighting conditions, screen flicker rates, and extended hours in front of the screen.*

To avoid eyestrain try simple exercises like scanning objects in the room to increase eye flexibility and palming (placing your palms over your eyes for complete darkness for 15-20 seconds) to relax your eyes.

Avoid Inner Aisles

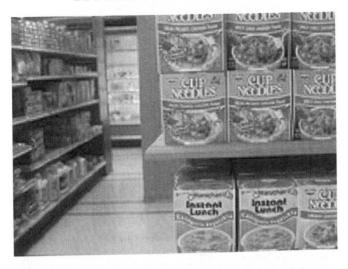

Have you ever noticed that the outside aisles at a grocery store are healthier than the inner aisles? The outside aisles contain mostly fresh fruits, vegetables, dairy products, meats, and other natural foods. The more you move inward, the more processed the food becomes. Go for the "clean burning" foods. Foods on the outside aisles usually have less than 5 ingredients and no preservatives making them a better choice!*

Stick to the outer aisles and take advantage of these "clean burning" foods. You will find fresh and healthy selections to add to your lifestyle.

Overcome Fear with Faith

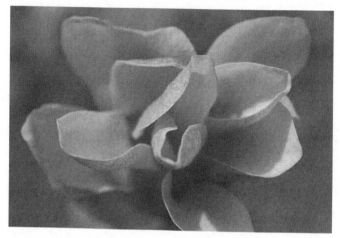

"When you face the future, what do you see? Do you look at it with eyes of doubt? Do you expect the worst? The way to overcome our fears is to proclaim your faith. Our faith is what allows us to enter the future - not with a question mark, but with an exclamation point!"

Do you have fear now? Just believe that it will all be fine and just go for it!

Do the Right Thing

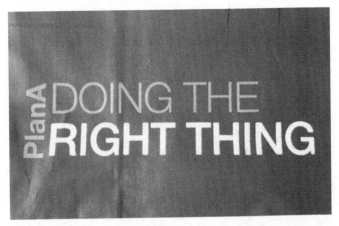

"In a moment of decision the best thing you can do is the right thing. The worst thing you can do is nothing." - Theodore Roosevelt

All successful people are decisive when it comes to making a decision. Sometimes we feel like avoiding the issue and moving on. We all know what the right thing is. We just need to do it.

Tea Tree Oil for Smelly Feet

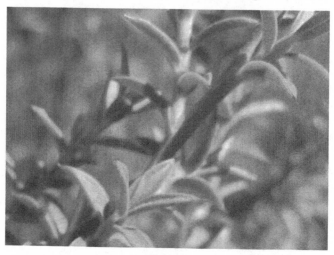

Foot odor is embarrassing for anyone! At least one-third of people suffer from smelly feet. In such a fast-paced world, our feet work overtime. They are home to 250,000 sweat glands, which can produce around one cup of sweat per day. Since our feet live in shoes, the sweat cannot evaporate as it does on the rest of our body. Sweat is used to regulate our body temperature and mix that with the bacteria growing on our feet and you have a bad odor.*

Tea Tree Oil is a great antifungal and antibacterial remedy. Add 5 to 10 drops of tea tree oil to warm water in shallow pan and soak your feet for 10 - 15 minutes nightly. You can also add tea tree foot powder in your shoes too.

Dr. S. Don Kim

Avoid Hot Water
for Your Skin

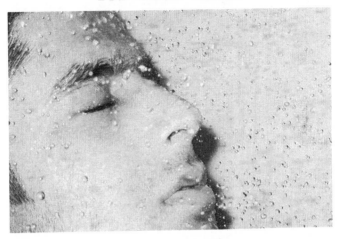

Hot showers can be a great relaxer, but it can strip your body of its natural oils! Start with that warm shower, but end with some cool water. The health benefits of taking cool showers are: better circulation as the cool water forces your blood to circulate back to your organs, better looking skin, in that it closes your pores after you cleanse, healthier hair as it gives it a nice shine, as well as some mental benefits in waking you up and getting energized.*

Take that warm shower, but circulate that with some cool water! It's a great way to get energized in the morning as well as a fresh new look each day.

Refined Sugar and Minerals

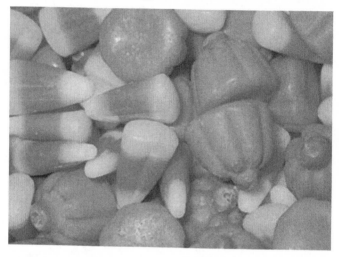

Refined sugars can wreak havoc on a healthy lifestyle, but did you know it has many other significant consequences? Here are just a few to know: Sugar can suppress your immune system, it can upset the mineral relationships in your body causing chromium and copper deficiencies, it can cause a rapid rise in adrenaline as well as anxiety, sugar causes loss of tissue elasticity and function, it can weaken eyesight, it causes premature aging, and it contributes to obesity.*

Think about your sugars! You might think they're great for satisfying in the moment, but they'll do more damage in the long run.

Count Your Blessings

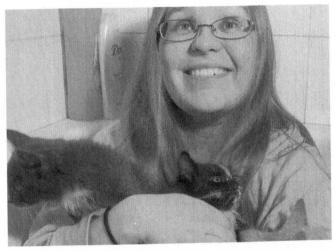

If you tend to focus on the negative side of things, you're not doomed to carry a cloud over your head for the rest of your life. Even the most committed pessimist can learn the skill of optimism.

It's simple. Count Your Blessings. While pessimists tend to focus on what is wrong with their lives, optimists are more likely to count their blessings.

Benefits of Mangoes

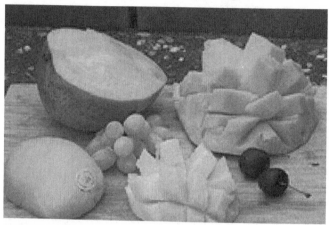

The mango is a powerhouse in fighting against free radicals that cause cancer. One small mango provides a quarter of your recommended daily allowance of vitamin C, two-thirds of your daily quota of vitamin A, with an abundance of vitamin E and fiber. They are also rich in vitamin K, phosphorous, magnesium, potassium and beta-carotene. Mangoes are also noted as being a "high volume" food, meaning you get a lot of food for only 135 calories.*

Stock up on your antioxidants and go grab some mangoes. They make an excellent refreshing snack during your day!

Are You Limping out of Bed in the Morning?

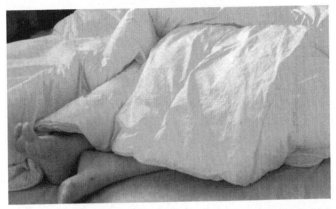

Do you have pain when you first put your heel down on the floor in the morning? You might have a heel spur or plantar fasciitis. It is caused when the plantar fascia (the dense strip of tissue that helps support the arch of the foot) undergoes force from the weight of the body. Over time, this causes stress and tears on the plantar fascia where it attaches to the heel bone. When the body tries to repair itself it will try to attach the fascia to the heel bone, which could cause bone spurs.*

If this pain comes daily for at least a week without improvement, you need to see your foot doctor. Aggressive stretching and bracing can save you from long invasive treatments of this problem.

Junk Food Drains Your Body

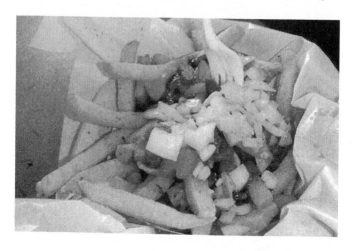

"Garbage In - Garbage Out!" If only it was that simple. Since junk food has few nutrients, your body has to use it's own nutrients to help digest the food. With the addition of dyes and chemicals, our bodies use even more of their stored resources to detoxify what was just taken in. How productive is that in our health? When we eat refined sugar our immune system is compromised by almost 50%. Our bodies resources are better used to keep us healthy not to detoxify and digest the junk we consume.*

Steer away from the drive-thru! Take a few extra moments in the morning to pack yourself a healthy snack and lunch for the day. Pack it with nutrients so your body can work for you!

Increase Your Metabolism by Lifting Weights

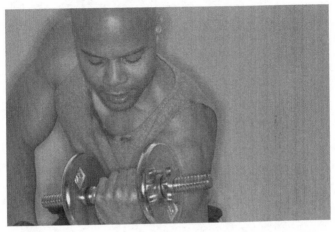

Resistance training is very important in your daily exercise routine, but did you know that it also speeds up your metabolism? In certain cases, for every pound of lean muscle you create, you can count on losing an extra 35-50 calories per day, up to 1,500 calories a month, or up to 18,000 calories per year while resting. That means that while you're at rest, you could be losing an extra 5 pounds of body fat.*

Add lifting weights to your exercise routine and watch your body work to tone and bump up your metabolism. It's the workout that continues after you've left the gym.

Healthy Cooking Oil

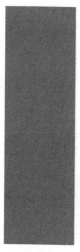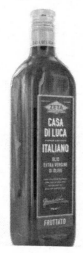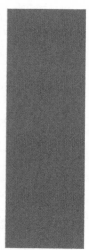

It's not about eliminating fat from your diet, it's about getting smart about the good fats you should keep in your diet. "A combination of monounsaturated fats (olive and peanut oil), polyunsaturated fats, and saturated fats (coconut and palm oil) is the best." When purchasing cooking oils look for the phrasing "cold pressed" or "expeller pressed" to make sure you are getting undamaged oils. Oils are fragile and heat or chemical processing will damage their properties.*

In the grocery store, look for cooking oils in tinted dark bottles. It's more than nice packaging; the dark bottles are keeping the oils safe from heat and light damage.

Don't Give Up!

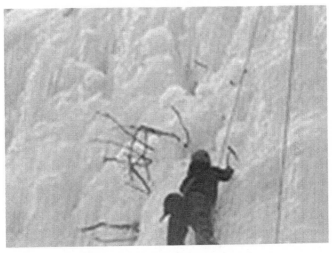

"Many of life's failures are people who do not realize how close they were to success when they gave up." - Thomas Edison

You may be a lot closer to success than you realize. When you feel like giving up, remember that each failure is getting you one step closer to success!

Prevent Gout with Cherries

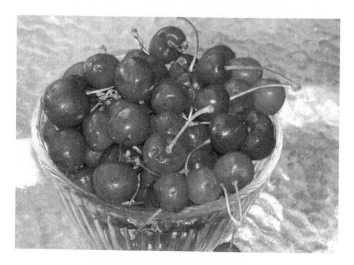

To reduce or even eliminate gout pain, try fresh cherries! Fresh cherries have great anti-inflammatory properties that help reduce gout and even arthritis pain. Gout is caused by the rise of uric acid levels in your body and the simple consumption of fresh, tart cherries, which have the fighting power of anthocyanins, will reduce these levels thus eliminating gout. Tart cherries have also been known to aid in muscle pain and sleep disorders.*

Pick up some organic concentrated cherry juice or some dried cherries. They make a great addition to your meals and they will be a natural way for you to relieve pain in your body.

Get an Exercise Buddy

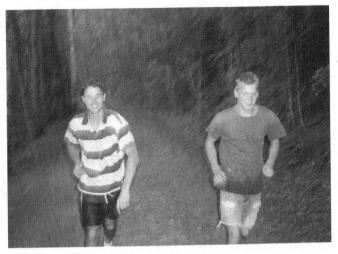

Exercise is a great way to keep healthy, but it's also hard to do it by yourself. Fitness experts say that having an exercise buddy will keep you more focused on your goals and it will make the time more fun instead of like work. Another benefit happens outside of the gym. If your health goals include eating healthier, an exercise buddy will help you by keeping you accountable on your eating habits and will join you in them so you're not alone.*

Find an exercise buddy! They will help you through this long, hard process to help you become a better and healthier you!

Relax with Lavender Oil

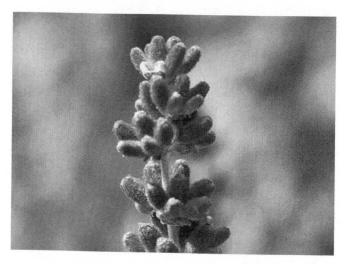

Lavender oil is great for aromatherapy, but did you know that it has many other health benefits? It helps in treating migraines, headaches, anxiety and depression; it helps induce sleep, it's a pain reliever, it can stimulate urine production, it aides against respiratory problems such as throat infections, the flu and cough. It's also used in hair care, improving blood circulation; it treats indigestion, it's great for immunity, and skin care.*

Go get yourself some lavender oil. If you're feeling stressed, place 3 drops of pure lavender oil on a soft cloth and inhale deeply.

Go for Garlic

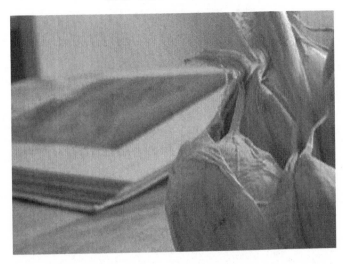

An apple a day keeps the doctor away...the same goes for garlic! Garlic has been known as a natural "cure-all." Garlic has great antioxidant and blood cleansing properties; it is also great for cardiovascular health and high cholesterol. Garlic has 1% of the potency of penicillin that makes it a great antibiotic and unlike other antibiotics; bacteria cannot develop a resistance against it. Two-three cloves of garlic can help prevent a cold, but don't take too much as it can irritate your digestive system.*

Add garlic to your meals and enjoy the health benefits. Remember to not microwave garlic as it kills the active ingredients!

Be Open for Feedback

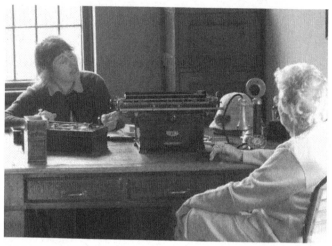

"Feedback is the breakfast of champions" - Rick Tate

Whatever you are doing or plan on doing, ask for feedback from people around you. You will be glad you did!

Home Remedies for Heel Pain

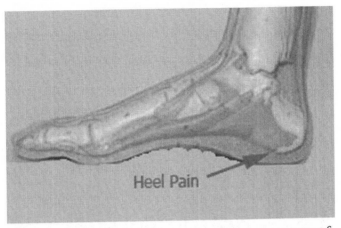

Heel Pain

Plantar fasciitis is the most common cause of heel pain. You might notice it when you take your first step in the morning or when you run, walk, hike or just after a long workday. Plantar fasciitis is an inflammation of the fascia (a long ligament at the base of the foot). Here are some tips to aide in heel pain: decrease your activity to low intensity, ice massage your arch and heel with a frozen water bottle, try heel lifts to take pressure off the arch, use a night splint to stretch your plantar fascia, get custom orthotics or supportive shoes and remember to STRETCH!*

Don't ignore heel pain! If the condition is untreated, small micro tears can develop that could lead to developing heel spurs or deterioration of the plantar fascia.

Incredible Benefits of Live Food

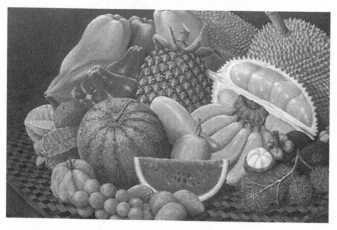

Living foods are those that contain enzymes, which assist in the digestion of foods. They have been called the "life force" and "energy" of food. We need enzymes to absorb all the good nutrients that food can give us. "All cooked food is devoid of enzymes, furthermore cooking food changes the molecular structure of the food and renders it toxic." A lifestyle of eating live foods will help increase your energy, aide in digestion as well as giving you a "light" feeling instead of the heavy after meal feeling most people get.*

Maximize the food you love and gain ALL of the health benefits. Living foods have higher nutrient values and that's great for your body and mind!

Your Own Massage Oil

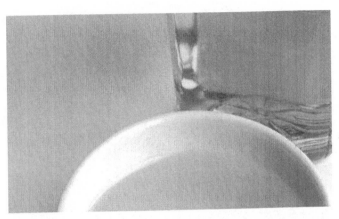

Everyone loves a good massage at the end of a long workday. Make your own massage oil at home! Tailor made to exactly what you want and need...and it's easy! You will need 6 teaspoons of a carrier oil and 8 drops of an essential oil. Carrier oils help dilute the highly concentrated essential oils so they can be used for massage. Good carrier oils are: sweet almond, grapeseed, canola, safflower, sunflower, sesame, wheat germ, olive and peanut oil. Add in an essential oil, like eucalyptus, to help relieve muscle aches and pains.*

Go to the store and grab some oils! Make your own and share with friends.

More Fish in Your Diet

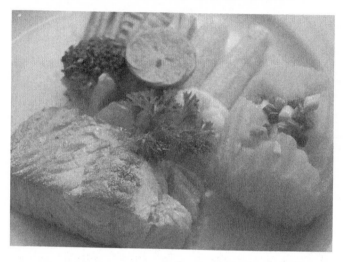

Fish is a high-protein and low-fat food that gives your bodies the great health benefits of omega-3s. These fatty acids provide our bodies with the following benefits: they help maintain cardiovascular health, they are important in prenatal and postnatal neurological development, they reduce tissue inflammation, they reduce the symptoms of rheumatoid arthritis, they can reduce depression and halt the mental decline in aging generations as well as play a role in aiding cardiac arrhythmia.*

Let's get more omega-3s! Try fish for dinner a few nights a week instead of the traditional chicken or beef. Your family will love the change and the benefits!

Amazing Benefits of Foot Reflexology

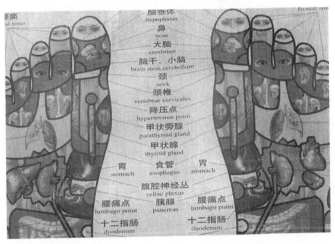

Relaxation, improved blood circulation, pain reduction, regularity, improved memory and improved relationships! These are just a few of the amazing benefits of foot reflexology. The foot is a great hub of nerves that affect your entire body. Foot reflexology is based on the function and activity of these reflexes throughout your whole body. When these reflexes are stimulated it can bring about physiological changes that benefit your health and everyday living!*

Look for a foot reflexology clinic and experience this amazing therapy for your overall health.

Amazing Health Effects of Honey

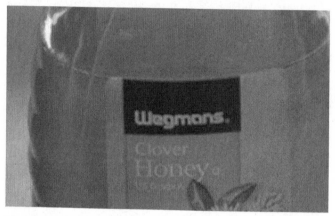

Honey can be used as a sweetener, an energy source, used for weight loss, improving athletic performance, a great source of vitamins and minerals, as well as having antibacterial and antifungal properties, and is a great source of antioxidants. Mixing some honey with milk and using it as a facial mask will help smooth and soothe your skin. Honey is also great for healing wounds as it stimulates the wound tissues.*

Grab some organic honey from your store and take advantage of the many ways honey can benefit your life!

Dr. S. Don Kim

Don't Get Stuck in Front of Your Computer

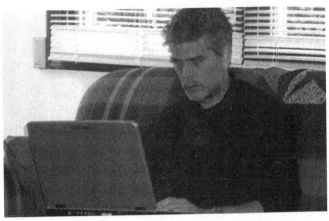

Are you experiencing back and neck pain while at work? Computer related pain is very common. Here are some tips to help alleviate some of the problems: keep good posture because when you start to slouch your muscles will shorten and become very tight. Make sure your keyboard and mouse are positioned so your elbows are at a 90-degree angle. Your monitor should be at eye level or just below to alleviate neck pain.*

Don't stay in front of computer for more than 30 minutes at a time. Walk around and stretch often. Raise both arms up in the air then pull them down behind your neck squeezing your scapular bones. You need to fight your posture going forward with this exercise.

Are You Happy Inside?

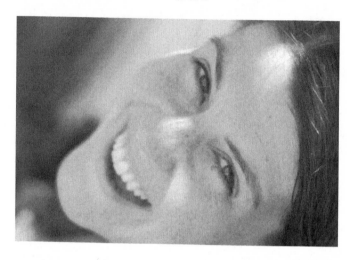

Happiness is an inside job! If you can't find happiness inside yourself you'll never find it in the outside world, no matter where you move. Wherever you go, there you are. You take yourself with you. If you're happy inside then you live in paradise no matter where your residence is.

Are you happy inside? Do one thing today that will make you say "yes" to that question.

Increase Mitochondria to Burn More Fat

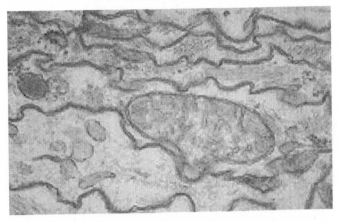

Mitochondria produce energy in your cells. When you increase the number of mitochondria in your cells you are turning up your body's power to burn calories and fat. To help raise the number of mitochondria, you need to exercise regularly. Don't forget to cool off because it will help the mitochondria increase in size and numbers.*

Try swimming, rowing or just walking! They raise your heart rate gradually and use major muscle groups that cause a greater demand in energy production thus creating more mitochondria.

Watch out for
Raynaud's Disease

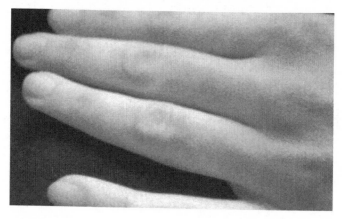

Raynaud's is caused by a vasospasm, a decreased blood flow to the tips of the fingers or the toes. You may have swelling, itching, discoloration, redness, or pain. Women are more susceptible to this condition. About 5 percent of Americans have Raynaud's disease and 40 percent of this group has their toes affected. Cold or stress can trigger the disease causing the skin to turn white or blue. In severe cases it can develop into skin sores or gangrene from continuous attacks.*

Improve your circulation by exercising. It's important that you wear the right shoes and insulated socks to protect yourself from the cold. You can also use heat packs behind your knees to improve circulation to your toes.

Pack Before You Overeat

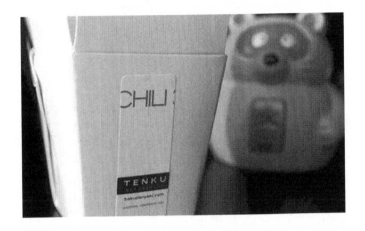

Practice your portion control! Eating out is fun, but it can cause havoc on your body from over-eating and all the extra calories. Remember a few simple tips and you can relax a little more at the table. If you're eating out with a loved one, try sharing an entrée. Most restaurants will split the dish onto two separate plates so it looks more appealing. Also, ask for a to-go box right away! Packing half your meal will save you from overeating and give you some great food the next day.*

Strategize before you order! You don't have to skip the entrée you want, just pack half of it away for tomorrow or share it with a loved one! It's that easy.

Do You Have Sleep Apnea?

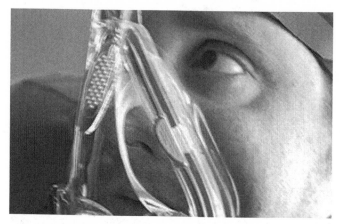

Sleep Apnea affects around 30 million Americans and millions more are at risk for the illness. Obstructive sleep apnea is the periodic cessation of breathing while asleep. It is caused by blockage of the airway by the tissues in the back of the throat. Sleep apnea can cause heart disease and stroke. Cardiac arrhythmias and congestive heart failure are also much more common among sleep apnea sufferers. It has increased risk of diabetes and obesity, also problems such as headaches, poor exercise tolerance, hypertension, memory loss, stroke or heart attack, and lung disease.*

If you have symptoms, get tested for sleep apnea. A CPAP machine could help you breath at night. But you need to lose weight, avoid alcohol and sedative drugs.

Life is an Echo

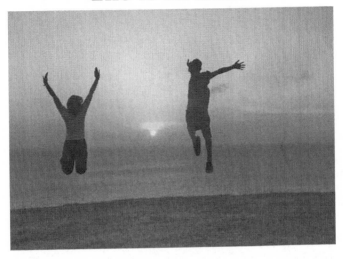

*"Life is an echo; what you send out comes
back."*
- Chinese Proverb

Send wonderful words, thoughts and love out
into the world and enjoy the echoes!

Enjoy Dark Chocolate

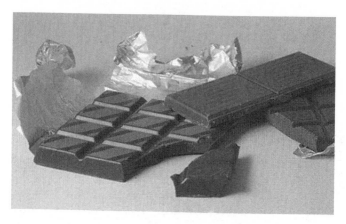

Cocoa in the dark chocolate has abundant poly-phenols called flavanol. It helps reduce blood pressure by relaxing arteries. It improves insulin sensitivity by decreasing fasting insulin and glucose levels. Cocoa flavanols have been shown to lower inflammation in tissues throughout the body, including pain and allergic reactions. And chocolate's potent antioxidants shield the endothelial cells lining the arteries as well as LDL cholesterol against free radical damage. Most importantly it makes you feel good by producing a sensation of pleasure in your brain.*

High-quality dark chocolate is sold in health food, specialty, and grocery stores. Look for bars that contain 70 percent cocoa or more. Limit your intake to no more than 25-50 g, or one quarter-half of a large bar, daily.

Stretch to Eliminate Heel Pain

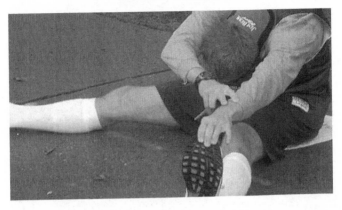

Around 10% of Americans suffer from heel pain. Those first steps in the morning can be very painful for those that do. Studies have shown that those who did stretching showed a 75 percent chance of having absolutely no pain. Sit with one leg crossed over the other, and stretch the arch of the foot by taking one hand and pulling the toes back toward the shin for a count of 10. Repeat 10 times, and perform at least three times a day*

Before you get out of bed, remember to stretch! Before you sit for long periods of time, remember to stretch! Today - remember to stretch!

Don't Eat from a Bag, Box, or Bucket

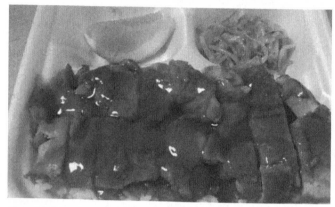

Snacking can be healthy, but also dangerous. When going for a snack, plate it up! Don't eat straight out of the bag, box, or bucket because you never see how much you actually eat. Place a portion on the plate, seal the bag, and then go enjoy your snack.*

Pre-portion and plate your snacks! Eating out of the bag, box or bucket is blind eating that only leads to excess calories.

Replace Sugar with Xylitol

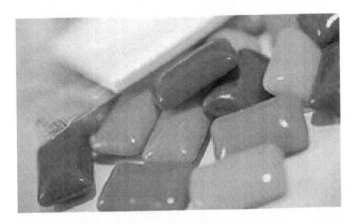

Did you know that "the body changes sugar into 2 to 5 times more fat in the bloodstream than it does starch?" That's one out of many reasons to find a sugar substitute. Xylitol is a natural substance that is found in many fruits and vegetables. Our bodies produce 15 grams of it daily during metabolism. Xylitol is a great sugar substitute because it has a glycemic index of 7, it has a minimal effect on blood sugar and insulin levels (making it great for diabetics), it also inhibits plaque and dental cavities by 80 percent and promotes tooth enamel.*

Try a little xylitol today! It's a great sugar substitute for cooking and baking. Besides the health benefits, it could save you a bit on the dentist bill as well!

Schedule Regular Vacations

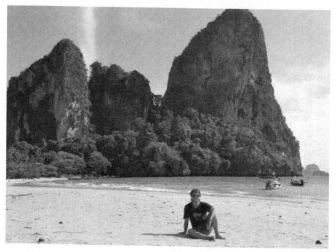

Vacations get shoved aside when other important things come up. Your regular vacations should be one of your priorities in life. Vacations have the following health benefits when taken regularly: they help us reconnect with ourselves and promote creativity, they allow for relaxation that can save us from burnout, we can "recharge our batteries," they help restore quality of sleep and mood, they can strengthen bonds, they relieve stress, and overall promote a better quality of life.*

Schedule regular vacations and commit to follow through! Your body and family will thank you for the benefits.

Strength Training Boosts Metabolism

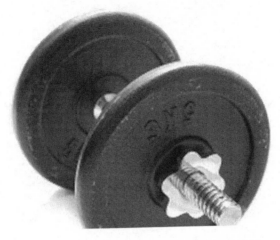

We have all heard that strength training can boost your metabolism. As we age, metabolism takes a dive and it becomes very important that we keep up a strength training routine. Think about this: each pound of muscle added during strength training will burn 50 calories a day. In other words, mere existence of muscles will burn more calories and keep you thinner!*

Add some muscles to burn more calories and boost metabolism! Strength training will ensure strong and thin body for many years to come.

Dark Room for Good Sleep

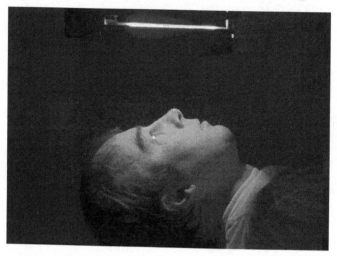

Sleeping in a dark room does more than give you some good beauty rest. Research has shown that children who sleep in a completely dark room are less likely to develop myopia, or nearsightedness. Even those that slept with a simple nightlight had a higher percentage of developing myopia. Research also shows that women who stay up late, work late hours, or sleep with the light on are at a higher risk of developing breast cancer because the light exposure at night interferes with the hormone melatonin, which aids against cancer.*

Sleep in a completely dark room and set a routine! Your body will get the rest it needs, which will help you stay healthy!

Make a Contract with Yourself

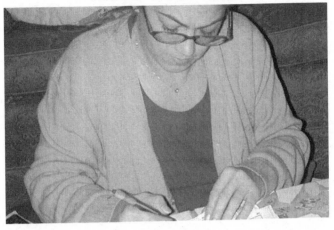

Making a contract with yourself tells those around you that you are making a commitment to a healthier you. The actual signing of the contract is not just a piece of paper with a state- ment of intent, it's a document that makes the situation real and forces you to be accountable for yourself! You wouldn't break a contract with a friend or colleague, so why would you break one with yourself? It's a reminder to keep your word, work hard, and see a healthy life become a reality!*

Make a contract with yourself! It's just a simple contract stating your goals and how you need to do them. Don't cheat yourself! Take the next step to a healthier you!

More Bowel Movement

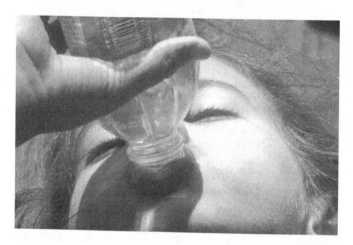

It's a common question: how many bowel movements should I have? In most cases, the average person should have at least one to two bowel movements a day. Healthy bowel movements are essential for optimal health because they eliminate undigested food and other waste materials. Having unhealthy bowel movements, or straining, can lead to blood in your stool or hemorrhoids. Some tips for healthy bowel movements are: regular exercise, drinking plenty of water, adding fresh fruits and vegetables to your diet, fiber, and avoid stress!*

Take care of your colon with these tips and you'll have better and healthier bowel movements. It's a health goal to take seriously!

Walking on a Marble

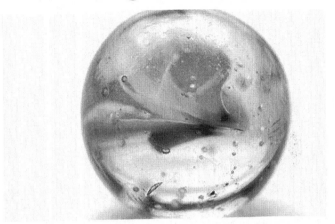

Walking on a marble is how people describe having a neuroma. A neuroma is a benign tumor that is made up of swollen and inflamed nerve cells located between the bones of the second and third toes on the ball of your foot. It is caused by compressing the "nerve of sensation between the ends of the metatarsal bones at the base of the toes." Symptoms of a neuroma are a sharp burning pain in the affected area as well as tingling when the foot is squeezed. The pain can also spread to the other toes making it difficult or painful to walk.*

If you are experiencing these symptoms, go to your doctor and get diagnosed. You can also prevent a neuroma by wearing custom orthotics, massaging your feet and wearing roomy comfortable shoes.

Burning Between the Toes

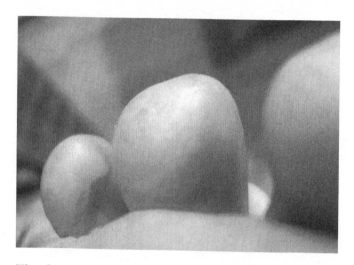

The formation of corns can be extremely painful and they can affect your every day life. The soft corn, or interdigital corn, forms between your toes often in pairs facing each other and are caused by the area taking in a lot of moisture causing a sore. These corns can give a burning sensation between the toes.* They are often caused by bones rubbing against each other also.

Find a good comfortable pair of shoes with larger toe box to avoid soft corns from forming. If you need a corn patch, watch out for those that contain acid because they will kill the corn, but they'll eat away the good skin around it too.

Ask This Question to be Healthy Naturally

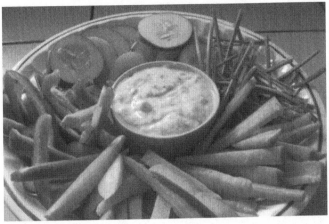

If you are interested in achieving optimal health, pay attention to the quality of food you eat! The closer the food is to its natural state, the better it will be for your body!

Always ask this question before you eat: "Is this food natural or man made?" If it is man made, avoid it at all costs. You are natural, so keep what goes into your body as natural as you can.

Potassium Iodide for Radiation Exposure

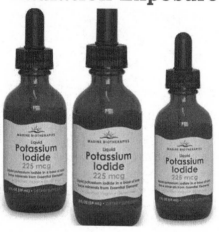

The recent earthquake and tsunami in Japan caused many explosions at nuclear reactors releasing radiation into the atmosphere. There have been concerns on where the radiation is going and whom it will affect. For those that have been affected, potassium iodide is given to help prevent thyroid cancer. It is a form of salt that protects the thyroid gland from radiation. It is most effective when given before exposure as it protects for about 24 hours.*

If you or someone you know lives within a 10-mile radius of a commercial nuclear plant, a stockpile of potassium iodide would be wise to have. It can be found online or at some health food stores.

Increase Omega 3 with Flaxseeds

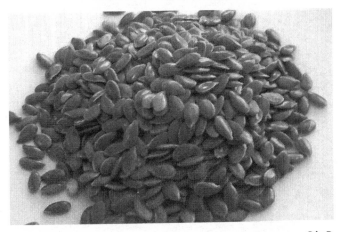

Trying to increase your intake of Omega 3's? Flaxseeds are a great choice and a good alternative if you are not a fan of cold-water fish. You can add flaxseed to your diet by either purchasing flaxseed oil or using the whole seed. By using the whole seed you add to your diet protein: fiber, minerals, phytochemicals (such as lignan), and omega 3's. Lignan is also believed to have anti-bacterial, anti-fungal, anti-viral and anti-cancer properties. 100 grams of flaxseeds will produce 26 grams of protein and fiber!*

Grind up some flaxseeds and add them to your cereal, salads, or any other food you like. They don't have a strong taste and they add a great crunch to any meal!

Kingdom of Health

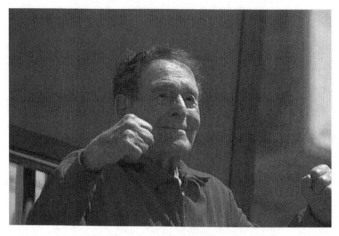

"Those who begin to exercise regularly and replace white flour, sugar, and devitalized foods with live, organic natural foods begin to feel better immediately. Exercise is king, nutrition is queen - put them together and you've got a kingdom."
- Jack LaLanne

Jack LaLanne was an American fitness, exercise and nutritional expert who recently passed away at the age of 96! He was also at least 50 years ahead of his time when he preached this lifestyle change. He will truly be missed. Let's all live the lifestyle that Jack preached!*

Obesity and Aging

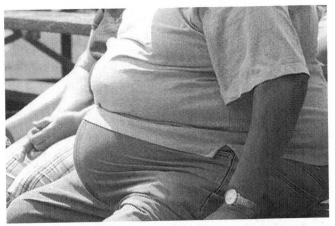

Being obese has the same effect as smoking in terms of premature aging. About one-third of American adults are considered obese! Obesity can take as many as 10 years off your life, which is the same as if you were a lifelong smoker. Even adults who were only 40 pounds over-weight could be losing as many as three years off their life. Obesity causes premature aging issues such as heart disease and stroke by rising blood pressure, unhealthy blood cholesterol and the development of diabetes.*

Nutrition and exercise are the most fundamental ways to keep our bodies healthy and yet they are the first to go to save a little time. Stop creating opportunities that take from your life and start living healthy to add to your life!

75% of Nail Salons Don't Properly Disinfect

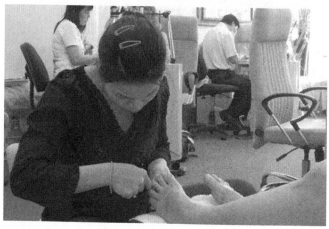

According to Podiatrist Dr. Robert Spalding, author of "Death by Pedicure," he states that "at this time, an estimated one million unsuspecting clients walk out of their chosen salon with infections - bacterial, viral and fungal." There is always a risk of infection when you visit a nail salon. It's possible to get cut and not even know it! And if you think about how they never turn customers away, whether they are sick or have an infection, you could easily catch something.*

Watch out for the cleanliness at your nail salon! Don't be afraid to ask about their disinfecting procedures or you could even bring your own instruments to the salon.

Just Do It

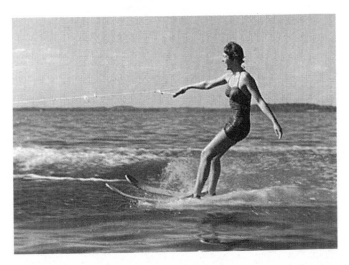

In old age, people are usually sorry for the things they did not do rather than for the things they did do.

If you are contemplating whether to do something or not, just do it! You will regret less later on!

Homemade Popsicles

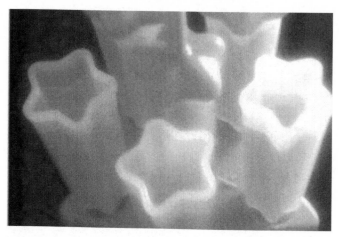

The weather is warming up and that means summertime treats! Homemade popsicles are a great and inexpensive treat that has many benefits. Besides being a very cool tasty treat, homemade popsicles help eliminate trash; by reusing molds instead of sticks, they are very healthy when you use organic fruits and vegetables, you can use leftover fruits and vegetables by freezing them and eliminate waste, they save money and they're great entertainment for kids AND adults!*

Buy a few popsicle molds and look for great healthy recipes. They'll be a treat everyone can enjoy when the weather warms up!

Dr. S. Don Kim

Eat Breakfast to Stay Sharp and Alert

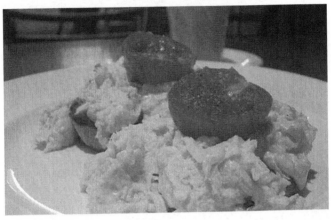

Breakfast is a vital part to the start of your day. Research has shown that people who take the time to have a good breakfast have more energy, improved concentration and performance, more strength and endurance, as well as helping to maintain weight control and low cholesterol levels. Breakfast is extremely vital to children before a day at school. It gives them better concentration, problem-solving skills and hand-eye coordination in the classroom, and improved performance on the playground.*

Don't skip breakfast for that quick coffee and pastry. Take the time to make yourself a full healthy meal and watch as you become a more sharp and alert you!

Progress, Not Perfection

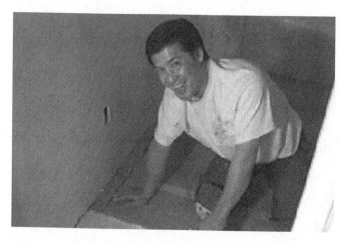

When changing your lifestyle habits from unhealthy habits to healthy habits, focus on progress, not perfection.

Don't be discouraged if you are not making big progress. Small changes will add up to be great later on! You will never be perfect, so just focus and appreciate the small progressions you make daily.

Do You Have a Flat Tire?

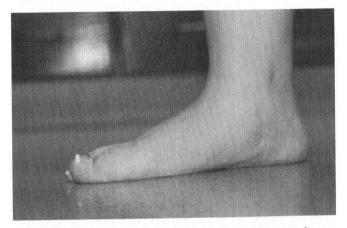

Think of your feet as tires to a car. If you have a flat tire you can't go anywhere and if you have a flat foot you can't really go anywhere either. Flat feet, or over pronation, is caused by weakened muscles due to heavy strain, such as standing or walking for long periods of time, aging and wearing shoes without proper arch support. When you have a flat foot, your foot shifts pressure to other parts of you foot causing pain and more serious problems such as heel spurs, ankle sprains, hip and lower back pain, and arthritis.*

If you have flat feet you need to see a podiatrist to evaluate a pair of custom made orthotics that would be helpful. A good pair of orthotics will help balance your whole body from your feet up!

Substitute for Soda Pop

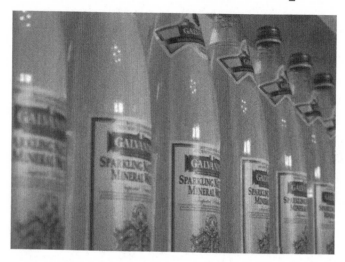

Want to kick the soda habit and take out all those extra calories during the day? Try making your own "soda alternative" by combining two simple ingredients: freshly squeezed juice and sparkling mineral water. Sparkling mineral water provides hydration to the body without the added sugar or calories. Pair that with some freshly squeezed oranges or berries and you have a great alternative to soda that won't pack in those extra calories.*

Next time reach for the fresh fruit and sparkling mineral water instead of the pack of soda on sale at the grocery store! It's a great summertime drink!

Be Kind

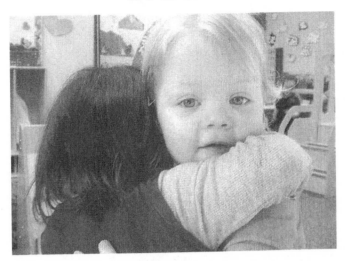

"Kindness is more important than wisdom, and the recognition of this is the beginning of wisdom"
- Theodore Isaac Rubin

Be kind to someone today. Try kinder words, a kinder gesture, a kinder smile. How do you feel now?

Wash Raw Vegetables with Vinegar

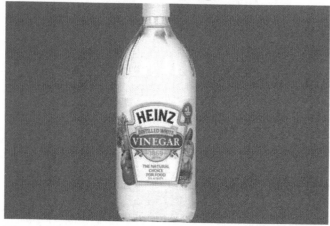

There's no more need for the expensive vegetable washes! You can make your own using a spray bottle, white vinegar and water. For hard-skinned fruits and vegetables: fill the bottle with equal parts of white vinegar and water and then spray your produce rubbing in the mixture and then rinsing. For soft-skinned fruits and vegetables: fill a bowl with equal parts of white vinegar and water and then soak your produce for a minute and then rinse. The acid in the vinegar kills off the bacteria, wax and pesticide residue found on most produce.*

Try this all-natural and inexpensive wash to make sure your vegetables are clean and healthy for your body!

Natural Facial Treatment

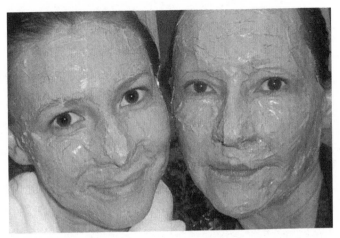

Homemade, natural facial treatments are inexpensive and most of the ingredients are in your home already. For example, here's a natural face-lift recipe that helps fight fine lines and wrinkles. The ingredients: 2 egg yolks and 1 teaspoon of sugar. That's it! Whisk the egg yolks until they are firm and consistent. Add the sugar gradually and mix well. Apply to face and leave on for 25 minutes. Wash off with warm water using a washcloth. Eggs are rich in protein albumin and amino acids that tone the skin and smooth out lines.*

Take a look in the pantry and try making your own facial masks! It's inexpensive, safe, natural, and wonderfully healthy!

Achilles Tendonitis

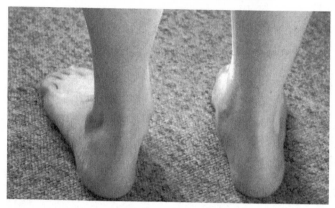

Achilles Tendonitis affects the large tendon in the back of the ankle through inflammation and irritation. This condition is most common in athletes who do not warm up properly and if not treated immediately can lead to pain and swelling. The most common causes of Achilles tendonitis are lack of flexibility and overpronation. A major symptom associated with this condition is pain in the back of the heel right above where the tendon attaches to your heel. This pain usually occurs after inactivity, such as getting up in the morning. Treatment is as simple as resting the tendon to relieve the inflammation.*

Rest and stop all activities that aggravate the tendonitis for 2-4 weeks. Try shoe inserts. Stretch the tendon 10 counts, 10 repetitions, three times per day. Use a towel or a belt to stretch the tendon while sitting.

Dr. S. Don Kim

How to Combat Constipation

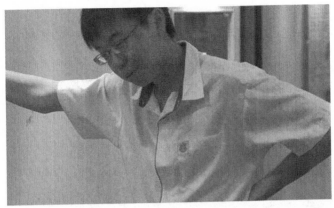

Constipation can happen occasionally or for some, a lot more than they want. There are some simple things you can do everyday to make sure you have great digestive health. First thing is that you must always try to eat regular meals and keep them on time instead of on the run! Take a look at the foods you eat and choose a healthy diet for healthy digestion. Drink lots of fluids throughout the day and pay attention to your body's signals. Exercising and making a schedule to get organized can reduce constipation and stress.*

Always check with your doctor if you are having troubles with constipation. Take a look at your lifestyle and see what your body is saying about it.

Physical Activity and the Brain

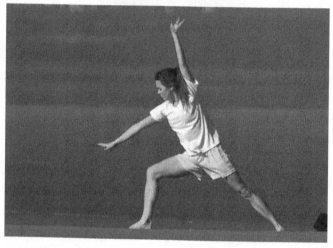

Losing weight has many different factors and one of them is appetite control. It's the Achilles heel of weight loss. New studies have shown that exercising can actually help curb your appetite through the hypothalamus gland. The hypothalamus gland is responsible for your hunger and appetite control by monitoring food intake and energy requirements. Physical activity has been shown to help reduce the appetite stimulating hormones found in the hypothalamus.*

Get active! Physical activity has long been known to be a brain stimulator and when we give our bodies healthy activity, our brains will send the same healthy message back to our bodies!

Popeye's Mighty Spinach

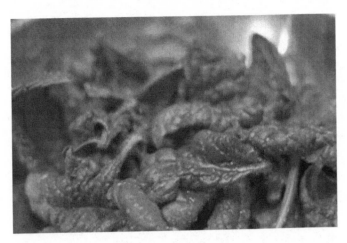

Spinach is one of the most nutritious foods out there! Spinach has cancer-fighting antioxidants, it improves cardiovascular health, it fights against ovarian and prostate cancers, it improves brain function and even protects against aging. Just think, one cup of spinach contains more than your daily need of vitamin K and vitamin A, almost all of the folate and manganese your body needs and 40 percent of your need of magnesium. It's also the source of more than 20 different nutrients such as dietary fiber, calcium and protein.*

Grab some spinach! It's a great nutritional choice that packs a lot of health benefits without all the extra calories.

Become a Person of Success

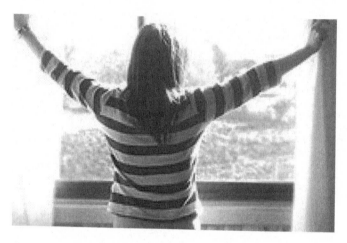

"Success is not to be pursued; it is to be attracted by the person you become." - Jim Rohn

Become a better person everyday in every aspect of your life. Become a better father, a better mother, a better son, a better daughter, a better worker, a better friend and a better spouse. You will become more successful in no time!

Dr. S. Don Kim

Go Barefoot on Soft Surfaces

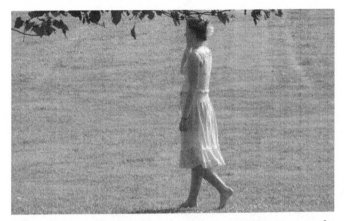

It's time to take off the shoes! According to studies, going barefoot "develops muscle strength in the feet, legs, and hips which are usually used less rigorously when locked up in restrictive shoes." You will also stretch and strengthen calf muscles, improve your form, agility and equilibrium. Go bare-foot, but keep it soft and start slow! Look for places like golf courses, athletic fields, parks, and beaches. Walk a few minutes a day as your feet strengthen and get used to the feeling. As they strengthen, increase your time and enjoy the benefits of being barefoot.*

Take off your shoes after a long day at work and walk on a soft surface. Remember to keep your feet safe from sharp objects, use sunscreen when outside, and listen if you start to feel any pain.

1MWellness.com

Sources

Page   * Reference | Photo credit

4   http://www.mayoclinic.com/health/flatfeet/DS00449/ DSECTION=symptomsome | Photo | Day 8 | by Perfecto Insecto on Flickr | used under a Creative Commons Attribution license

5   http://www.allaboutwater.org/water-facts.html | Pouring water portrait | Photo | © 2009 Philppe Put | used under a Creative Commons Attribution-No Derivative Works license

6   http://www.calciuminfo.com/osteperosis/calciumdeficiency.aspx | Photo | Wet Broccoli | by Robert Carboneau on Flickr | used under a Creative Commons Attribution-Share Alike license.

7   http://www.cascadebloodcenters.org/about_blood/components.htm | Photo | Leafy green | by Ben Lancaster | used under a Creative Commons Attribution license

8   http://www.americanheart.org/presenter.jhtml | Photo | Salmon – Makoto, Sydney AUD3 | by Alpha on Flickr | Used under a Creative Commons Attribution Share Alike License

9   http://www.cancersalves.com/articles/Microwave.html | Photo | Microwaving an egg | by Denise Chan | Used under a Creative commons Attribution Share Alike license

10   http://www.encyclopedia.com/doc/1G1-114477556.html | Photo | 40+60 Feet, Euw. | by bark on Flickr | Used under a Creative Commons Attribution License

11   Alexander, Rick. Victory Over Fat: Six Steps to Permanent Fat Loss and Super Health. Galahad, 2005. 135. | Photo | Food and Drink: Water (fizzy) | by Adam Raoof | Used under a Creative Commons Attribution License

12   Pratt, Steven and Kathy Mathews. Superfoods Rx. HarperCollins, 2003. | Photo | a little of everything good | by EvelynGiggles on Flickr | Used under a Creative Commons Attribution License

13   Trenev, Natasha. Probiotics: Nature's Internal Healers. Avery, 1998. | Photo | "Natural" with Kiwi and Raspberries, Mmm. | by Silus Grok | Used under a Creative Commons Attribution Share Alike license

14   http://webcache.googleusercontent.com/search?q=cache:LH4--171gmEJ:www.usuhs.edu/fap/resources/ le/FootInjury.ppt+bodyweight+pressure+foot+site:.edu&cd=3&hl=en&ct=clnk&gl=us Photo | Socks and Shoes | by Ben Babcock | Used under a Creative Commons Attribution License

15   Margel, Douglas. The Nutrient-Dense Eating Plan. Basic Health Publications, 2005. 162. Photo | Salt and Pepper in Sausalito | by smi23le on Flickr | Used under a Creative Commons Attribution License

16   Dreyer, Danny and Katherine Dreyer. Chi Walking. Simon and Schuster, 2006. Photo | Group walking along the Los Gatos creek trail | by Don DeBold | Used under a Creative Commons Attribution License

17   "Power Naps Can Increase Alertness, Mood." Apples for Health.

http://www.applesforhealth.com/HealthySenior/pnciam10.html. Photo | Power Nap Now | by Tony Bowden | Used under a Creative Commons Attribution Share-alike license

18   Kurzweil, Ray and Terry Grossman. Fantastic Voyage: Live Long Enough to Live Forever. Rodale, 2004. Photo | Johannes Eats Pumpkin Curry | by avidd on Flickr | Used under a Creative Commons Attribution License

19   Fields, Jonathan. "Why 99.9% of Your Ads Will Never Be Seen." http://www.jonathanfields.com/blog/why-999-of-your-ads-will-never-be-seen/ Photo | Rainbow | by Richard North | Used under a Creative Commons Attribution License

20   http://www.cbsnews.com/stories/2010/01/20/health/healthy_living/main6119907.shtml. Photo | Couch Potato | by Richard Summers | Used under a Creative Commons Attribution license.

21   http://www.cbsnews.com/stories/2010/01/20/health/healthy_living/main6119907.shtml. Photo | Kiwanja Kenya Calling | by Ken Banks | Used under a Creative Commons Attribution license.

22   The Chemical Sunscreen Health Disaster. http://www.skinbiology.com/toxicsunscreens.html. Photo | Stephen Applying Suntan Lotion | by Tom Hodgkinson | Used under a Creative Commons Attribution Share Alike license

23   Photo | IMG_9077 | by Lucy Boynton | Used under a Creative Commons Attribution License.

24   Photo by Linds :)|flickr.com.

25   Understanding Brain Damage and Endocrine Disorders Caused by MSG. http://www.truthinlabeling.org/Dang.html. Photo | Monosodium Glutamate Crystals | by Sage Ross | Used under a Creative Commons Attribution Share Alike license.

26   http://www.huffingtonpost.com/dr-rock-positano/ankle-sprains-are-notorio_b_219652.html. Photo | Ankles | by Paul Huxley | Used under a Creative Commons Attribution license.

27   Beck, Melinda. "Defending Against Disease--With Vitamin D." Wall Street Journal Online. http://online.wsj.com/article/SB121607103504852163.html. Photo | Old Woman | by Ed Yourdon | Used under a Creative Commons Attribution Share-alike License.

28   Mech, Susan Delaney. "Rx for Quilters." C&T Publishing, 2000. 97. Photo | Chocolate | by John Loo | Used under a Creative Commons Attribution License.

29   "Health Benefits of Citrus Fruits: Oranges, Grapefruits, Lemons and Limes." http://www.steadyhealth.com/articles/Health_Benefits_of_Citrus_Fruits__Oranges__Grapefruits__Lemons_and_Limes_a1141.html. Photo | "If you're looking for oranges on an apple tree..." | by turtlemom-4bacon on Flickr | Used under a Creative Commons Attribution Share-alike License.

30   "French Paradox." http://en.wikipedia.org/wiki/French_Paradox. Photo | Eiffel Tower | by Lodewijk Gelauff | Used under a Creative Commons Attribution Share-alike License.

31   Flemin, Jill. "How to Eat Like a Thin Person." LaCrosse Tribune. 29 Dec. 2009. http://www.lacrossetribune.com/article_87cca5f8-f48d-11de-a778-001cc4c03286.html. Photo | breakfast: menemen | by Paul Keller | Used under a Creative Commons Attribution License.

32   [http://volleyball-base.com/blog/2008/01/14/to-brace-or-not-to-brace-that-is-the-question. Photo | Sprained Ankle | by kkrn | Used under a

Creative Commons Attribution License
33   Photo | Listen to your Mother | by Lisa C. Sjolund | Used under a Creative Commons Attribution License.
34   Borchard, Therese. "7 Healthy Reasons to Cry Your Eyes Out." http://www.beliefnet.com/Health/2009/04/How-Crying-Can-Be-Healthy.aspx. Photo | Crying is Okay Here | by misocrazy on Flickr | Used under a Creative Commons Attribution License.
35   "Dangers of Aspartame Poisoning." http://www.sweetpoison.com/aspartame-information.html. Photo | Soda Can Angle 1 | by yaybiscuits123 on Flickr | Used under a Creative Commons Attribution License
36   "How to Sweat for Detox." http://health.amuchbetterway.com/how-to-sweat-for-detox/

Photo | Sweat or rain? | by Kullez on Flickr | Used under a Creative Commons Attribution License
37   Laskawy, Tom. "New Research: Fructose Increases Risk of Diabetes, Heart Disease." http://www.grist.org/article/draft-new-research-links-high-fructose-corn-syrup-and-diabetes-heart-diseas/. Photo | No Sugar Added | by Peter Krefting | Used under a Creative Commons Attribution Share-alike License.
38   http://www.emedicinehealth.com/ingrown_toenails/article_em.htm. Photo | Toe nails have to be cut sometime...| by Victor Martinez | Used under a Creative Commons Attribution License
39   Kokoska, Robert. "Calorie and Meal Shifting ...." American Chronicle. http://www.americanchronicle.com/articles/view/120170. Photo | Salad | by Charles Haynes | Used under a Creative Commons Attribution Share-alike License.
40   Photo | by Sandy Richards.
41   "Diet of Walnuts, Blueberries Improves Cognition; May Help Maintain Brain Function." http://www.sciencedaily.com/releases/2007/11/071106122843.htm. Photo | Walnuts | by Pauline Mak on Flickr | Used under a Creative Commons Attribution License.
42   Quirino, Cory. "Avocados help prevent cervical cancer." http://showbizandstyle.inquirer.net/lifestyle/lifestyle/view/20090608-209438/Avocados-help-prevent-cervical-cancer. Photo | Avocado | Chad Miller | Used under a Creative Commons Attribution License
43   Photo | Mom Smiling Bench | by Dieu Pham | Used under a Creative Commons Attribution License.
44   "Should You Walk 10,000 Steps Per Day for Fitness?" http://walking.about.com/od/measure/f/10000steps.htm. Photo | Walk up Stairs | by Dan Eckert | Used under a Creative Commons Attribution License
45   Adams, Mike. "Secrets of Soil Nutrition." Natural News. http://www.naturalnews.com/020072.html. Photo | Vitamins! | by Bradley Stemke | Used under a Creative Commons Attribution License
46   http://health.nytimes.com/health/guides/disease/gout-chronic/causes-and-risk-factors.html Photo | Cherries | by David Wright | Used under a Creative Commons Attribution License
47   Nasal Irrigation." http://altmedicine.about.com/cs/allergiesasthma/a/SinusIrrigation.htm Photo | by Quinn Dombrowski on Flickr | Used under a Creative Commons Attribution Share-alike License
48   Kreydin, Amy. "Environment Benefits of Salt Lamps." http://

greenliving.suite101.com/article.cfm/salt_lamps. Photo | Salt Lamps made of Iranian salt | Arash Razzagh Karimi | Used under a Creative Commons Attribution License

49   Michrowski, Andrew. "Electromagnetic Pollution." http://www.consumerhealth.org/articles/display.cfm?ID=19990303163909 . Photo | Fatty watching himself on TV | by cloudzilla on Flickr | Used under a Creative Commons Attribution License

50   Photo | Cleaning the Attic | by Joe Shlabotnik | Used under a Creative Commons Attribution License.

51   http://www.ithaca.edu/faculty/nquarrie/contrast.html. Photo | Giant Bathtub | By Erica Nicol | Used under a Creative Commons Attribution Share-alike License.

52   http://www.abc-of-hiking.com/hiking-health/blisters.asp. Photo | White Socks in the Sun | by andy_5322 on Flickr | Used under a Creative Commons Attribution Share-alike License.

53   http://www.wellbeingjournal.com/index.php?option=com_content&task=view&id=92. Photo | Go ahead, jump! | by Robert S. Donovan on Flickr | Used under a Creative Commons Attribution License

54   http://informahealthcare.com/doi/abs/10.1517/13543784.12.7.1189. Photo | Mushrooms | by Mixer1 | Used under a Royalty Free License.

55   Photo | I Want to Hold Your Hand | by Kate Ter Haar | Used under a Creative Commons Attribution License.

56   http://webcache.googleusercontent.com/search?q=cache:XywXtfvb_PcJ:www.laskerfoundation.org/awards/2008_c_presentation.htm+Thirty+million+Americans+spent+%2434+billion+on+cholesterol+lowering+drugs+in+2009.&cd=8&hl=en&ct=clnk&gl=us&client=firefox-a. | Photo | Pills 3 | by e-Magine Art | Used under a Creative Commons Attribution License

57   Photo | Facial Massage | by o5com on Flickr | Used under a Creative Commons Attribution License.

58   http://www.japmaonline.org/cgi/content/abstract/94/3/261. Photo | Worn Out Shoes | by Ed Schipul | Used under a Creative Commons Attribution Share-alike License.

59   http://www.naturalnews.com/026579_risk_health_mercury.html. Photo | Nuts! | by Iain Buchanan | Used under a Creative Commons Attribution License

60   Photo | Handshake | by Miki Yoshihito | Used under a Creative Commons Attribution License.

61   http://www.alzheimersprevention.org/intro_4_pillars.htm. Photo | Old Couple | by Ian MacKenzie | Used under a Creative Commons Attribution License.

62   Photo | CityYear folks help out at tree planting | by Sodexo USA | Used under a Creative Commons Attribution License.

63   http://www.anniesremedy.com/herb_detail2.php. Photo | Aloe Aloe Aloe | by Garry Knight | Used under a Creative Commons Attribution Share-alike license.

64   http://www.livestrong.com/article/68749-compression-socks-work/. Photo | Ultimate Running Sock: right foot left foot | by Lululemon Athletica | Used under a Creative Commons Attribution License

65   Photo | ||||| | by Rodrigo Esper | Used under a Creative Commons Attribution License.

66   http://www.nlm.nih.gov/medlineplus/ency/article/000230.htm.
Photo | Feeling Fat | by Caitlin Regan | Used under a Creative Commons
Attribution License

67   Photo | Love Yourself | by Quinn Dombrowski | Used under a
Creative Commons Attribution Share-alike license.

68   http://life-enhancement.com/article_template.asp?ID=914. Photo |
Cinnamon Sticks | by S. Diddy | Used under a Creative Commons Attribution
License.

69   Photo | Another To-Do List | by whatleydude | Used under a Cre-
ative Commons Attribution License.

70   http://www.thirdage.com/foot-health/foot-problems-could-you-be-
wearing-the-wrong-shoes-0 . Photo | Keep or not? | by Kristin Kokkersvold |
Used under a Creative Commons Attribution License.

71   http://www.webmd.com/food-recipes/features/health-benefits-of-
green-tea. Photo | morning green tea | by Kanko* on Flickr | Used under a
Creative Commons Attribution License.

72   Photo | Laughing | by Quinn Dombrowski | Used under a Creative
Commons Attribution Share-alike license.

73   http://www.mayoclinic.com/health/red-wine/HB00089. Photo |
grapes | by Zest-pk on Flickr | Used under a Creative Commons Attribution
License.

74   Photo | The Way is Unclear | by Brent Newhall | Used under a
Creative Commons Attribution License.

75   http://abcnews.go.com/Health/Healthday/
story?id=4509945&page=1. Photo | Mike-baird-knee | by Mike Baird | Used
under a Creative Commons Attribution License.

76   http://www.sixwise.com/newsletters/05/06/22/the-major-health-
benefits-of-going-barefoot-really.htm. Photo | Sand on strain | by Arne Hjorth
Johansen | Used under a Creative Commons Attribution Share-alike License.

77   Photo | Pat on the back | by Jessie Terwilliger | Used under a Cre-
ative Commons Attribution license.

78   http://www.news-medical.net/news/20100118/Sunlight-and-vita-
min-D-deficiency-linked-to-17-varieties-of-cancer.aspx.
Photo | Me laying in the sun | by Deana Hunter | Used under a Creative Com-
mons Attribution License.

79   Photo | saturated writing| by tnarik / Eduardo on flickr | Used under
a Creative Commons Attribution Share-alike License.

80   http://www6.miami.edu/ummedicine-magazine/fall2005/fstory4.
html. Photo | handful of drugs | by Philippa Willitts on Flickr | Used under a
Creative Commons Attribution License.

81   Photo | Toe Art…Concern & Care | by Vinoth Chandar | Used
under a Creative Commons Attribution License.

82   http://www.reflexologychart.info/history.html. Photo | Tennis Balls
| by Atomic Taco on Flickr | Used under a Creative Commons Attribution
Share-alike License.

83   http://ods.od.nih.gov/factsheets/chromium.asp. Photo | Sugar | by
Uwe Hermann on Flickr | Used under a Creative Commons Attribution Share-
alike license.

84   http://www.cancer.org/Cancer/CancerCauses/OtherCarcinogens/
MedicalTreatments/menopausal-hormone-replacement-therapy-and-cancer-
risk. Photo | Gargar fanning herself | by TheSharpteam on Flickr | Used under

a Creative Commons Attribution Share-alike license.

85 Photo | Raking Leaves | by Aine | Used under a Creative Commons Attribution Share-alike license.

86 http://www.healthyeatingclub.org/info/articles/Minerals/iodine.htm. Photo | Tyler Kooper | by Jason O'Halloran | Used under a Creative Commons Attribution Share-alike license.

87 http://www.bodyecology.com/07/01/11/benefits_of_beneficial_bacteria.php. Photo | CreativeTools.se | by Creative Tools | Used under a Creative Commons Attribution License.

88 http://www.mayoclinic.com/health/first-aid-blisters/WL00008. Photo | Bacon-aid | by Florian Boyd | Used under a Creative Commons Attribution Share-alike License.

89 Photo | Messy bench-center | by David.R.Carroll | Used under a Creative Commons Attribution License.

90 http://www.aafa.org/display.cfm?id=9&sub=20&cont=285. Photo | Strawberries | by Sancho McCann | Used under a Creative Commons Attribution License.

91 Photo | Smelling the roses | by SamD2 on Flickr | Used under a Creative Commons Attribution License.

92 http://www.wrongdiagnosis.com/o/osteoarthritis/prevalence.htm. Photo | Cherries | Benson Kua | Used under a Creative Commons Attribution Share-alike License.

93 http://www.thesneakychef.com. Photo | Veggie Still Life | by Matchstick | Used under royalty free license.

94 http://www.nlm.nih.gov/medlineplus/athletesfoot.html. Photo | My sad right foot | by Chris Baranski | Used under a Creative Commons Attribution License.

95 Photo | Butterfly | by Fox_kiyo | Used under a Creative Commons Attribution Share-alike license.

96 http://www.intelihealth.com/IH/ihtlH/c/9339/31561.html. Photo | After drunken night at Chris' | by D. Sinclair Terrasidius | Used under a Creative Commons Attribution License.

97 http://lpi.oregonstate.edu/infocenter/vitamins/fa. Photo | Asparagus | by Farmer's Market | Used under a Creative Commons Attribution License.

98 Photo | 1 of 2 delightful girls give thumbs up | by Mike Baird | Used under a Creative Commons Attribution License.

99 http://www.medicinenet.com/tongue_problems/article.htm. Photo | Tongue | by nathamnac87 on Flickr | Used under a Creative Commons Attribution License.

100 http://www.foot-pain-explained.com/bursitis.html. Photo | hold them | by Victor Bezrukov | Used under a Creative Commons Attribution License.

101 Photo | Dirt Road and Wooden Fence, Plezenti Village, Buzau County, Romania | by Gabriel | Used under a Creative Commons Attribution License.

102 Photo | Gift | by Asenat29 on Flickr | Used under a Creative Commons Attribution License.

103 http://www.migraines.org/treatment/treather.htm. Photo | I just want the white ones! | by Quinn Dombrowski | Used under a Creative Commons Attribution Share-alike license.

104 Photo | These are a few of my favorite things | by Conor Ogle |

Used under a Creative Commons Attribution License⌐¬¬.

105   http://www.umm.edu/altmed/articles/raynauds-phenome-non-000140.htm. Photo | Not quite at home in the snow | by Micah Ogle | Used under a Creative Commons Attribution License.

106   http://faculty.ncwc.edu/ddaley/B231n%20Integument.htm. Photo | Kitchen Window | by Dominic Alves | Used under a Creative Commons Attribution License.

107   Photo | Best Friends Forever| by Don LaVange | Used under a Creative Commons Attribution Share-alike license.

108   http://www.epa.gov/iaq/pubs/insidest.html. Photo | Home Depot Tropical Room | by Λ VV Λ on Flickr | Used under a Creative Commons Attribution Share-alike license.

109   http://www.mgwater.com/calmagab.shtml. Photo | Green Soybeans| by Kanko | Used under a Creative Commons Attribution License.

110   http://www.foothealthfacts.org/Content.aspx?id=1483. Photo | Soccer Training | by Tommy Wong | Used under a Creative Commons Attribution License.

111   Photo | Crossing the Finish Line | by slgckgc on Flickr | Used under a Creative Commons Attribution License.

112   http://www.emedexpert.com/tips/music.shtml. Photo | Lianne Asleep | by Richard Riley | Used under a Creative Commons Attribution License.

113   http://www.webmd.com/asthma/allergy-asthma-proof-home. Photo | Making the bed | by Melissa Gutierrez | Used under a Creative Commons Attribution Share-alike license.

114   Photo | "ghar" Mountain | by DVIDSHUB on Flickr | Used under a Creative Commons Attribution License.

115   http://shoeallergies.50webs.com/allergy.htm. Photo | Contact Dermatitis | by Digitalgadget at en.wikipedia | Used under the Public Domain.

116   http://jnci.oxfordjournals.org/content/91/20/1751.full. Photo | Untitled | by Procsilas Moscas | Used under a Creative Commons Attribution License.

117   http://jnci.oxfordjournals.org/content/92/1/61.full. Photo | Tomato Soup | by Madzia Bryll | Used under a Creative Commons Attribution License.

118   http://www.webmd.com/fitness-exercise/features/how-to-look-thinner-instantly. Photo | Standing Tall 2008 | by Marion Doss | Used under a Creative Commons Attribution Share-alike license.

119   Photo | Heaven vs. Hell | by Ally Aubry | Used under a Creative Commons Attribution License.

120   http://www.mothernature.com/Library/Bookshelf/Books/47/64.cfm. Photo | Rome, Italy – Constantine's Stinky Foot and Steph | by Benjamin Vander Steen | Used under a Creative Commons Attribution License.

121   http://www.mayoclinic.com/health/cataracts/DS00050/DSECTION=causes.Photo | Colorful Fruit | by Justin | Used under a Creative Commons Attribution License.

122   http://www.antioxidants-anti-aging-super-foods.com/blood-clots.html. Photo | October 2010 | by Roberto Verzo | Used under a Creative Commons Attribution License.

123   http://www.ballroom-dancing-online.com/the-health-benefits-of-ballroom-dancing. Photo | Ballroom Dancing | by Nathan Meijer | Used under a Creative Commons Attribution License.

124   http://www.agingcare.com/Featured-Stories/139710/nutritional-drinks-seniors-elderly-problems.htm. Photo| Milk Bottle | by Nick Piggott | Used under a Creative Commons Attribution License.

125   http://www.yourfoothealth.com/haglunds-deformity.html. Photo | The price of wearing nice shoes | by Gunnar Grimnes | Used under a Creative Commons Attribution License.

126   Photo | Thursday Hang Around | by Daniel Giovanni | Used under a Creative Commons Attribution License.

127   Photo | 5/365 | by Anna Gutermuth | Used under a Creative Commons Attribution License.

128   http://www.helpguide.org/life/healthy_weight_loss.htm. Photo | Feet on Scale | Used under a Creative Commons Attribution share-alike License Wikipedia Commons.

129   http://www.rand.org/pubs/research_briefs/RB5018/index1.html. Photo | Kissing Couple | by Betacam | Used under a royalty free license.

130   http://www.acefitness.org/certifiednewsarticle/720/will-toning-shoes-really-give-you-a-better-body. Photo | by Lainee Richards

131   http://www.webmd.com/skin-problems-and-treatments/features/dry-skin-causes. Photo | dry | by Quinn Dombrowski | Used under a Creative Commons Attribution Share-alike license.

132   http://www.livestrong.com/article/158439-inversion-therapy-benefits. | Photo by Kim Perkins.

133   http://www.organicfacts.net/health-benefits/vegetable/health-benefits-of-sweet-potatoes.htm. Photo | Sweet Potato Pie | Tamara Polajnar | Used under a Creative Commons Attribution Share-alike license.

134   http://www.health.harvard.edu/fhg/updates/update0705c.shtml. Photo | Sauteed Spinach | by Laurel Fan | Used under a Creative Commons Attribution Share-alike license.

135   http://www.coachr.org/barefoot_running.htm. Photo | Two females jog barefoot on Morro Strand Beach | by Mike Baird | Used under a Creative Commons Attribution License

136   Photo | Camp Taji obstacle course | by The U.S. Army | Used under a Creative Commons Attribution License.

137   http://lpi.oregonstate.edu/infocenter/phytochemicals/isothio. Photo | Beetroot, Mozzarella, and Watercress salad | by Alpha | Used under a Creative Commons Attribution Share-alike license.

138   http://familydoctor.org/online/famdocen/home/common/digestive/disorders/087.html. Photo | Heartburn Info | by Everett Mar | Used under a Creative Commons Attribution License.

139   Photo | soccer practice | by woodleywonderworks on Flickr | Used under a Creative Commons Attribution License.

140   http://news.medill.northwestern.edu/chicago/news.aspx?id=170666&print=1. Photo | for love_yellow: Charles Jordan, Paris France Yellow Pumps | by Cheryl (Eraphernalia Vintage on FlickRiver) | Used under a Creative Commons Attribution Share-alike license.

141   http://www.stevia.com/Stevia_Article.aspx?Id=2413. Photo | Stevia | by onezzzart on Flickr | Used under a Creative Commons Attribution License.

142   http://www.everynutrient.com/healthbenefitsofcelery.html. Photo | Carrot, Celery, Spinach,Watercress Juice | by Tamara Smith | Used under a Creative Commons Attribution License.

143   Photo | Young Americans for Liberty War Protest on Tax Day | by Fibonacci Blue on Flickr | Used under a Creative Commons Attribution License.

144   http://fooddemocracy.wordpress.com/2007/11/09/chew-on-this-us-soda-consumption. Photo | Soda Cans | by nicoleleec | Used under a Creative Commons Attribution License.

145   http://www.usnews.com/science/articles/2010/11/10/fructose-poses-gout-risks-even-in-women.html?PageNr=2 . Photo | DSC03203 | by Alex Gorzen | Used under a Creative Commons Attribution Share-alike license.

146   http://www.bendigobank.com.au/public/generationgreen/sustain-able-living/work/plants-to-remove-toxins.asp. Photo | Milwaukee, Near South Side, Teweles Building 1918 | by Vincent Desjardins on Flickr | Used under a Creative Commons Attribution License.

147   http://www.sott.net/articles/show/170455-Avoid-Flu-Shots-Take-Vitamin-D-Instead]. Photo | Preparing the Injection 11-10-08 | by Steven Depolo | Used under a Creative Commons Attribution License.

148   http://www.quinoatips.com/quinoa-glycemic-index. Photo | Kale & Mushroom Quinoa | by Jennifer | Used under a Creative Commons Attribution License.

149   http://articles.mercola.com/sites/articles/archive/2010/11/19/vitamin-b12-helps-ward-off-alzheimers.aspx. Photo | Eggs of many colors | by WoodleyWonderworks | Used under a Creative Commons Attribution License.

150   http://www.bbc.co.uk/news/magazine-11790486. Photo | I love daddy's shoes! | by Zakwitnij!pl Ejdzej | Used under a Creative Commons Attribution Share-alike license.

151   http://articles.mercola.com/sites/articles/archive/2010/11/22/the-common-cold-simple-strategies-for-prevention-and-treatment.aspx. Photo | hydrogen peroxide | by Kelly Cree | Used under a Creative Commons Attribution License.

152   http://www.healingdaily.com/oral-chelation/mercury.htm. Photo | 31 with filling when I came in | by Eric Schmuttenmaer | Used under a Creative Commons Attribution Share-alike license.

153   http://www.podiatrym.com/letters2.cfm?id=39805&start=1 | ** http://www.chron.com/disp/story.mpl/health/7302429.html. Photo | 12/15/2006 – Pillz (darvocet) | by Amayzun | Used under a Creative Commons Attribution License.

154   http://www.worldhealthyfoods.com/pomegranates. Photo | Pomegranate | by Tony Hisgett | Used under a Creative Commons Attribution License.

155   http://www.stop-foot-pain.com/foot-facts.htm. Photo | Walk in Icho Namiki | by Jordi Sanchez Teruel | Used under a Creative Commons Attribution Share-alike license.

156   http://www.webmd.com/sleep-disorders/sleep-needs. Photo | Lose your sleep before your decision, not after it | by Scott McLeod | Used under a Creative Commons Attribution License.

157   http://www.drhotze.com/Dr-Hotzes-Wellness-Program/Bioidenti-cal-Hormones/Men.aspx. Photo | 24 | by Ben Newton | Used under a Creative Commons Attribution License.

158   http://www.webmd.com/balance/goji-berries-health-benefits-and-

side-e. Photo | Boxthorn| by Robin | Used under a Creative Commons Attribution Share-alike License.

159   http://www.raysahelian.com/massage.html. Photo | A Well Deserved Massage | by Joe Goldberg | Used under a Creative Commons Attribution Share-alike License.

160   http://health.howstuffworks.com/wellness/natural-medicine/home-remedies/home-remedies-for-foot-pain.htm. Photo | IMG_3437.JPG | by David Boyle | Used under a Creative Commons Attribution Share-alike license

161   http://www.ncbi.nlm.nih.gov/pubmed/20884921?dopt=Abstrac. Photo | All the Toothpaste you really need | by Kenneth Lu | Used under a Creative Commons Attribution License.

162   Photo | The McIntosh family at force | by Neil McIntosh | Used under a Creative Commons Attribution License.

163   http://www.lourdesnet.org/services/hyperbaric.php. Photo | n1521480092_30664132_2809 | by KOMUnews on Flickr | Used under a Creative Commons Attribution License.

164   http://news.yahoo.com/s/livescience/20101217/sc_livescience/peoplesnackmorewhoeatinfrontoftvcomputerscreens. Photo | eating lunch | by Michelle Morgan | Used under a Creative Commons Attribution License

165   http://www.medicalnewstoday.com/articles/204578.php. Photo | Walk | by Clarkston SCAMP on Flickr | Used under a Creative Commons Attribution License.

166   http://www.organicfacts.net/organic-oils/natural-essential-oils/health-benefits-of-peppermint-oil.html. Photo | peppermint | by Jill Robidoux | Used under a Creative Commons Attribution License.

167   http://www.mayoclinic.com/health/dehydration/SM00037. Photo | Luke is really thirsty | by Melissa Hughes | Used under a Creative Commons Attribution License.

168   http://www.livestrong.com/article/256945-is-eating-frequent-smaller-meals-better-for-weight-loss. Photo | Baby Spinach in Superior Stock | by Alpha | Used under a Creative Commons Attribution Share-alike license.

169   [http://www.healthcastle.com/energy_drinks.shtml. Photo | Top of Red Bull Can | by [F]oxymoron on Flickr | Used under a Creative Commons Attribution License.

170   http://www.mercolahealthyskin.com. Photo | lotion | by MountainMade WV Handmade Art | Used under a Creative Commons Attribution License.

171   http://www.articlesbase.com/shopping-articles/flat-feet-versus-fallen-arches-1023890.html. Photo | What's all the fuss about? | by Vivek Patankar | Used under a Creative Commons Attribution License.

172   http://www.livestrong.com/article/170506-benefits-of-black-cherry-juice. Photo | Black Cherries | by Market Manager | Used under a Creative Commons Attribution License.

173   http://www.dummies.com/how-to/content/following-a-cardio-plan-for-weight-loss.html. Photo | Barefoot in the Park | by lululemon athletica | Used under a Creative Commons Attribution License.

174   http://www.turningpointechiro.com/services.php?SERVICE=47. Photo | My orthotic shoe inserts | by Douglas Muth | Used under a Creative Commons Attribution Share-alike license.

175   http://www.medicalnewstoday.com/articles/203276.php. Photo |

Ballgame Grub | by Patrick W. | Used under a Creative Commons Attribution License.

176   http://www.seedsofdeception.com/Public/AboutGeneticallyModi-fiedFoods/index.cfm. Photo | Corn Field | by fishhawk on Flickr | Used under a Creative Commons Attribution License.

177   http://envirocancer.cornell.edu/Factsheet/general/fs42.bodytype.cfm. Photo | NASA technology could aid in the interpretation of mammograms | by NASA Goddard Space Flight Center | Used under a Creative Commons Attribution License.

178   http://abcnews.go.com/Health/ColdandFlu/exercise-stave-off-colds-infections/story?id=12135405. Photo | Wunder Groove Crop for Yoga | by lululemon athletica | Used under a Creative Commons Attribution License.

179   http://www.everydayhealth.com/health-report/dry-skin-relief/dr-wu-causes-of-dry-skin.aspx. Photo | Heater | by Steve Swayne | Used under a Creative Commons Attribution Share-alike license.

180   http://www.purposedrivenlife.com/en-US/AboutUs/AboutThe-Book/sampleChapters/chapter1.htm. Photo | If someone asks me why…| by Nick Bramhall | Used under a Creative Commons Attribution Share-alike license.

181   http://www.associatedcontent.com/article/372478/the_health_ben-efits_of_deep_breathing.html?cat=51. Photo | relax 2 | by Lululemon Athletica | Used under a Creative Commons Attribution license

182   http://www.healthy.net/scr/news.aspx?Id=10483. Photo | legs of a young man running | c cienpies.net | Used under a royalty free License.

183   http://www.livestrong.com/article/94116-burn-calories-day. Photo | Central Park – Nov 2008 – 12 | by Ed Yourdon | Used under a Creative Commons Attribution Share-alike license.

184   Photo | Sister's Love | by Carmella Fernando | Used under a Creative Commons Attribution License.

185   http://www.foot.com/info/cond_pregnancy_feet.jsp. Photo | 1 weeks to go woohoo! | by Nina Matthews | Used under a Creative Commons Attribution License.

186   http://www.vitalitymagazine.com/the_healing_art_and_science_of_qigong. Photo | Summary World Tai Chi & Qigong Day | by TarcisioTS | Used under a Creative Commons Attribution Share-alike license and the GNU Free Documentation License.

187   http://www.yogatuneup.com/blog/2010/08/25/yoga-therapy-cell-phone. Photo | MP4 | by Schnaibel | Used under a royalty free license.

188   http://www.associatedcontent.com/article/538479/15_health_ben-efits_of_beets_fight_cancer_pg2.html?cat=51. Photo | red beets | by Stacy Spensley on Flickr | Used under a Creative Commons Attribution License

189   http://www.fertilityauthority.com/blogger/cindy-bailey/2010/07/09/watch-out-organic-vs-natural-labeling. Photo | Are the stickers organic too? | by Andrew Hyde | Used under a Creative Commons Attribution License.

190   http://www.adeshoes.com/content/calluses. Photo | Zermatt- My feet after hiking | by Andrew Bossi | Used under a Creative Commons Attribution Share-alike license.

191   http://www.brighthub.com/health/diet-nutrition/articles/12822.aspx. Photo | Shopping center 3 | by Fish | Used under a royalty free License.

192   Photo | Hug Steve | by Bev Sykes | Used under a Creative Commons Attribution License.

193   http://today.msnbc.msn.com/id/6708310/ns/today-foodwine. Photo | Pete's BBQ – Mission District | by Michael McCauslin | Used under a Creative Commons Attribution License.

194   http://www.diabetes-guide.org. Photo | Day 248/365 – Fresh Veggies | by Anita Hart | Used under a Creative Commons Attribution Share-alike license.

195   http://stressfracturefoot.org. Photo | Soccer UD | by pnijhuis | Used under a royalty free License.

196   Photo | Baking Perfectionists? | by San Jose Library on Flickr | Used under a Creative Commons Attribution Share-alike license.

197   http://www.cancerproject.org/protective_foods/building_strength/iron.php. Photo | Roast Suckling Pig – Top – Cutler and Co AUD44 | by Alpha | Used under a Creative Commons Attribution Share-alike license.

198   Photo | Leading by Example | by The Mighty Tim Inconnu | Used under a Creative Commons Attribution License.

199   http://www.mayoclinic.com/health/trans-fat/CL00032. Photo | potato chips | by stu_spivack on Flickr | Used under a Creative Commons Attribution Share-alike license.

200   http://www.wikihow.com/Heal-a-Broken-Toe. Photo | In the examination room | by frankenstoen on Flickr | Used under a Creative Commons Attribution License.

201   http://www.webmd.com/vitamins-supplements/ingredient-mono-1172- KRILL%20OIL.aspx?activeingredientid=1172& activeingredientname= KRILL%20OIL. Photo | Krill Oil? | by Randal Cooper | Used under a Creative Commons Attribution Share-alike License.

202   http://www.articleswave.com/articles/negative-effects-of-television.html. Photo | Mom watches TV | by Goldemberg Fonseca de Almeida | Used under a Creative Commons Attribution license.

203   http://www.sheknows.com/health-and-wellness/articles/805434/how-protein-and-fiber-can-keep-you-satisfied. Photo | steaming | by miheco on Flickr | Used under a Creative Commons Attribution Share-alike License.

204   Photo | One BIG Sandwich | by Matthew Nuzum | Used under a Creative Commons Attribution License.

205   http://dermatechrx.com/athletesfoot. Photo | Show me the Bunny | by Wendy Harman | Used under a Creative Commons Attribution License.

206   http://www.pcrm.org/health/veginfo/vegetarian_foods.html. Photo | Oh yes. | by Robin Zebrowski | Used under a Creative Commons Attribution License.

207   http://www.sparkpeople.com/resource/nutrition_articles.asp?id=1485. Photo | My grocery list | by Ben Becker | Used under a Creative Commons Attribution License.

208   Photo | Lily of the Valley | by Leo Seta on Flickr | Used under a Creative Commons Attribution License.

209   http://www.suite101.com/content/looking-to-stay-healthy-try-a-health-food-store-online-a325766. Photo | Vegetables in Whole Foods Market | by Masahiro Ihara | Used under a Creative Commons Attribution License

210   http://www.everydayhealth.com/foot-health/toenail-cutting-tips.aspx. Photo | Polka Dotted Pedicure | by Jessie Terwilliger | Used under a Creative Commons Attribution License.

211   http://www.beauty-cosmetic-guide.com/beauty-sleep.htm. Photo | Sleeping | by RelaxingMusic on Flickr | Used under a Creative Commons

Attribution Share-alike License.

212   http://www.estheticiansalary.org/the-benefits-of-eating-a-high-fiber-diet.html. Photo | Salad | by Wendy | Used under a Creative Commons Attribution License.

213   http://www.organicfacts.net/nutrition-facts/seeds-and-nuts/nutritional-value-of-cashew-and-chestnut.html. Photo | Roasted Chestnuts – Squirrel's Nuts, Oakleigh AUD8.99 Per kg | by Alpha | Used under a Creative Commons Attribution Share-alike license.

214   http://foodsthatheal.blogspot.com. Photo | Shiitake Mushrooms | by frankenstoen on Flickr | Used under a Creative Commons Attribution License.

215   http://orthoinfo.aaos.org/topic.cfm?topic=A00163. Photo | Untitled | by Podma | Used under a Creative Commons Attribution License.

216   http://www.visionworksusa.com/computereyestrain.htm. | Photo | 40 + 28 Eye Strain | by bark on Flickr | Used under a Creative Commons Attribution License.

217   http://www.shapefit.com/perimeter.html. Photo | Untitled | by Ryan Dickey | Used under a Creative Commons Attribution License.

218   Photo | Happy Birthday – Magnolie – for my friend Raffael | by digital cat | Used under a Creative Commons Attribution License .

219   Photo | doing the right thing | by Clive Darr | Used under a Creative Commons Attribution Share-alike license.

220   [http://ezinearticles.com/?Smelly-Feet---Foot-Odor-Causes&id=923895.Photo | Tea Tree Leaves | by John Tann | Used under a Creative Commons Attribution License.

221   http://www.ineedmotivation.com/blog/2008/04/4-reasons-why-you-need-to-take-cold-showers/. Photo | self Portrait | by Gagneet Parmar | Used under a Creative Commons Attribution Share-alike license

222   http://doctorweightlossprogram.com/nutrition/668. Photo | Candy Corn and Candy Pumpkins closeup | by Juushika Redgrave on Flickr | Used under a Creative Commons Attribution License.

223   Photo | 20080921_9999_28b | by Sanna Pudas | Used under a Creative Commons Attribution License.

224   http://www.suite101.com/content/the-health-benefits-of-mangoes-a73235. Photo | Mango | by Tatiana Gerus | Used under a Creative Commons Attribution License.

225   http://www.eorthopod.com/content/plantar-fasciitis-heel-pain. Photo | feet in the morning | by Juan Antonio Flores Segal | Used under a Creative Commons Attribution License.

226   http://mystrategiclifeplan.com/lose-weight/articles/got-a-high-crap-diet. Photo | Ghetto Fries from Max's in Chicago | by Stu Baker | Used under a Creative Commons Attribution Share-alike license.

227   http://www.muscleandfitness.com/training/53. Photo | Man Lifting Weights | by Spirit-Fire on Flickr | Used under a Creative Commons Attribution License.

228   http://www.weightandwellness.com/smartfats.html. Photo | CreativeTools.se - PackshotCreator - Olive oil | by Creative Tools on Flickr | Used under a Creative Commons Attribution License.

229   Photo | Rojachergeist | by gego2605 on Flickr | Used under a Creative Commons Attribution Share-alike license.

230   http://ezinearticles.com/?Cherry-Juice-Helps-to-Fight-Gout-Pain-and-Reduce-Uric-Acid-Levels&id=3394422. Photo | cherries | by Bev Sykes |

1MWellness.com

Used under a Creative Commons Attribution License.

231   http://www.exercisefriends.com/info/detailednews. asp?NewsID=102. Photo | Kevin L, Wayne E. Running along trail | by Russ Brady | Used under a Creative Commons Attribution License.

232   http://www.organicfacts.net/organic-oils/natural-essential-oils/ health-benefits-of-lavender-essential-oil.html. Photo | Lavender | by Rutger | Used under a Creative Commons Attribution License .

233   http://naturalhealthremedies.org/what-are-the-health-benefits-of-garlic. Photo | Garlic | by David Pursehouse | Used under a Creative Commons Attribution License.

234   Photo | Black Country Living Museum – The Worker's Institute – desk | by Elliot Brown | Used under a Creative Commons Attribution License.

235   http://www.northcoastfootcare.com/pages/Heel-Pain-and-Plantar-Fasciitis.html. Photo | heel pain | by happyfeet34 on Flickr | Used under a Creative Commons Attribution License.

236   http://www.living-foods.com/faq.html. Photo | Tropical Fruits oil painting | by Wizan Zaini | Used under a Creative Commons Attribution License.

237   http://makeup.ygoy.com/bodycare/index.php. Photo | Rice Bran Oil | by Robin | Used under a Creative Commons Attribution Share-alike license.

238   http://www.notjustthekitchen.com/health-beauty/health-benefits-of-eating-fish. Photo | Salmon Stk. | by Pokkie | Used under the Public Domain.

239   http://www.livestrong.com/article/25602-benefits-foot-reflexology. Photo | Podographique | by Fred | Used under a Creative Commons Attribution License.

240   http://www.organicfacts.net/organic-animal-products/organic-honey/health-benefits-of-honey.html. Photo | Honey | by nanamin2003 on Flickr | Used under a Creative Commons Attribution License.

241   http://www.ehow.com/facts_6017930_computer-use-neck-pain. html. Photo | brian on computer | by Brian Kelley | Used under a Creative Commons Attribution Share-alike license.

242   Photo | Smile | by Romain Guy | Used under a Creative Commons Attribution Share-alike license.

243   http://www.weightlossforall.com/metabolism-raise-mitochondria. htm. Photo | Powerhouse | by Matthew Britton | Used under a Creative Commons Attribution License.

244   http://www.yourbodycanheal.com/raynaudsdisease.html. Photo | Raynaud's Phenomenon | by Michelle Tribe | Used under a Creative Commons Attribution License.

245   http://thehealthylivingsite.com/2010/06/23/easy-strategies-to-help-you-eat-less-and-prevent-overeating. Photo | Tenku Bankudenyaki in a takeout box | by Paul Joseph | Used under a Creative Commons Attribution License.

246   http://www.rjmatthewsmd.com/Definitions/obstructive_sleep_apnea%202.htm. Photo | 306/365 – and I need something more | by Robert Anthony Provost | Used under a Creative Commons Attribution License.

247   Photo | Jump for Joy | by Bing Ramos | Used under a Creative Commons Attribution License.

248   http://www.organicfacts.net/health-benefits/other/health-benefits-of-dark-chocolate.html. Photo | Dark Chocolate | by Simon A. Eugster | Used under a Creative Commons Attribution License.

249   http://www.sciencedaily.com/releases/2006/11/061101150739.htm.

Photo | Stretching | by Tony Alter | Used under a Creative Commons Attribution License.

250   http://www.rd.com/health/15-diabeticfriendly-snacks-tips. Photo | Chicken Plate Japanese Food | Michael Dorausch | Used under a Creative Commons Attribution Share-alike license.

251   http://www.naturalnews.com/022692.html. Photo | XylitolGum – 08 | by Kyle Lam | Used under a Creative Commons Attribution Share-alike license.

252   http://stress.about.com/od/workplacestress/a/vacations.htm. Photo | Yes.. I am a beach bum | by Davidlohr Bueso | Used under a Creative Commons Attribution License.

253   http://www.brighthub.com/health/fitness/articles/24734.aspx. Photo | Dumbbell | by Keith Ramsey | Used under a Creative Commons Attribution Share-alike license.

254   http://www.suite101.com/content/sleep-in-the-dark-for-better-health-a289667. Photo | Dark room Dream 6/52 | by Tom Hart | Used under a Creative Commons Attribution License.

255   http://www.drpeeke.com/web/page/616/sectionid/553/interior.asp. Photo | Xy Grades | by Bart Everson | Used under a Creative Commons Attribution License.

256   http://www.coloncleanseguide.com/articles/healthy-bowel-movement-how-to. Photo | Drink of Water | by Eden, Janine and Jim | Used under a Creative Commons Attribution License.

257   http://www.medicinenet.com/mortons_neuroma/article.htm. Photo | Marble | by Wolfgang Lonien | Used under a Creative Commons Attribution Share-alike license.

258   http://www.cornsontoes.com/treatment-for-corns. Photo | Burnt Toes | by Indi Samarajiva | Used under a Creative Commons Attribution License.

259   Photo | Roast Onion Dip + Veggies | by Theresa Carpenter | Used under a Creative Commons Attribution Share-alike license.

260   http://www.foxnews.com/health/2011/03/15/factbox-potassium-iodide-use-radiation-exposure. Photo | Glad to see Henry's isn't cashing in on the nuclear hysteria..oh wait | by Daniel | Used under a Creative Commons Attribution License.

261   http://www.care2.com/greenliving/how-to-increase-omega-3s-in-your-diet.html# Photo | Yellow Flaxseed | by Alisha Vargas | Used under a Creative Commons Attribution License.

262   http://en.wikipedia.org/wiki/Jack_LaLanne. Photo | Jack LaLanne | by Nathan Cremisino | Used under a Creative Commons Attribution Share-alike license.

263   http://www.usatoday.com/news/health/weightloss/2009-03-17-obesity-death_N.htm. Photo | Full Figured Man | by Tony Alter | Used under a Creative Commons Attribution License.

264   http://shine.yahoo.com/channel/beauty/6-things-your-nail-salon-doesnt-want-you-to-know-2469958. Photo | Pedicure 2 | by The Consumerist on Flickr | Used under a Creative Commons Attribution License.

265   Photo | Waterskiing on Lake Mendota | by uwdigitalcollections on Flickr | Used under a Creative Commons Attribution License.

266   http://www.growingagreenfamily.com/green-cooking-benefits-of-homemade-popsicles. Photo | Homemade Popsicles! | by Dana Robinson |

1M Wellness.com

Used under a Creative Commons Attribution Share-alike license.

267   http://www.webmd.com/diet/features/many-benefits-breakfast.
Photo | Parmesan Scrambled Eggs with Basil and Roasted Tomato | by Alpha |
Used under a Creative Commons Attribution Share-alike license.

268   Photo | Tom at Work | by Steven Burt | Used under a Creative
Commons Attribution Share-alike license.

269   http://www.footsmart.com/healthcondition.aspx?ailmentid=8.
Photo | Dr. Kim's Office.

270   http://www.examiner.com/healthy-living-in-minneapolis/healthy-
living-tip-substitute-mineral-water-for-soda. Photo | sparkling mineral water |
by avlxyz on Flickr | Used under a Creative Commons Attribution Share-alike
License

271   Photo | Hugging Friends | by Tom Trelvik | Used under a Creative
Commons Attribution Share-alike License.

272   http://frugalliving.about.com/od/cleaningtipsandrecipes/qt/Pro-
duce_Wash.htm. | Image by DL Hughes | Used under a Creative Commons
Attribution License.

273   http://www.skin-care-recipes-and-remedies.com. Photo | 100_9256
| by Neeta Lind | Used under a Creative Commons Attribution License.

**274   http://orthopedics.about.com/cs/ankleproblems/a/achilles.
htm. Photo | ankles | by Paul Huxley | Used under a Creative Commons
Attribution License.**

**275   http://www.getconstipationrelief.com/six-steps-to-combating-
occasional-constipation. Photo | wah...constipation | by Timothy Tsui |
Used under a Creative Commons Attribution Share-alike license.**

**276   http://www.livestrong.com/article/330484-the-hypothalamus-
gland-weight-loss. Photo | Girl doing exercises on Morro Strand State
Beach | by Mike Baird | Used under a Creative Commons Attribution
License.**

**277   http://www.livestrong.com/article/2700-facts-health-benefits-
spinach. Photo | Spinach | by Ted Major | Used under a Creative Com-
mons Attribution Share-alike license.**

**278   Photo | Open your wings | by A.M. | Used under a Creative
Commons Attribution License.**

**279   http://www.sheknows.com/health-and-wellness/articles/804306/
the-benefits-of-going-barefoot-and-tips-to-keep-your-bare-feet-safe.
Photo | Barefoot Lady | by Lee Haywood | Used under a Creative Com-
mons Attribution Share-alike license**

Dr. S. Don Kim

1MWellness.com

30562695R00189

Made in the USA
Middletown, DE
29 March 2016